Delicious Living

approved recipes
for people with type 2 diabetes
and everyone

Peter Howard

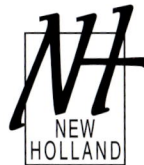

NH
NEW
HOLLAND

www.newholland.com.au

First published in Australia in 2006 by
New Holland Publishers (Australia) Pty Ltd
Sydney • Auckland • London • Cape Town

www.newholland.com.au
1/66 Gibbes Street Chatswood NSW 2067 Australia
218 Lake Road Northcote Auckland New Zealand
86 Edgware Road London W2 2EA United Kingdom
80 McKenzie Street Cape Town 8001 South Africa

National Library of Australia Cataloguing-in-Publication Data:

Howard, Peter, 1947- .
    Delicious living : approved recipes for people with type 2
    diabetes and everyone.

    Includes index.
    ISBN 9781741104356 (pbk.).

    1. Diabetes - Diet therapy - Recipes. 2. Diabetes. I.
    Title.

    641.56314

Publisher: Fiona Schultz
Production Controller: Linda Bottari
Project Editor: Michael McGrath
Designer: Karl Roper
Printer: SNP/Leefung Printing Co. Ltd. (China)

10 9 8 7 6 5 4

Contents

This book is dedicated to all people who have diabetes of all types,
to my supporters and folk who have been there for me all my professional life.

Peter Howard

This book was reviewed by Diabetes Australia Ltd's Health Care and Education Committee (HCEC)
in February 2006 and is endorsed for publication until February 2008.

A Message from Diabetes Australia

Being faced with the diagnosis of diabetes can be a great shock. Peter Howard is one of more than a million Australians who have had to come to grips with the news that they have a lifelong disease—for which there is currently no cure.

Clearly, diabetes cannot be taken lightly. It is a serious and complex condition that has reached epidemic proportions around the world. The good news, however, is that there are ways to effectively manage it so it doesn't interfere with the hopes, dreams and aspirations we hold for ourselves, our work and family lives.

Understanding is life's greatest ally, whatever the challenge we face. By providing accurate and up-to-date information, Diabetes Australia is committed to helping people with diabetes to face that challenge by being able to make well-informed choices.

Over the years, we have come to appreciate that people learn a great deal from others affected by diabetes, particularly about day-to-day issues that are so important to us.

Diabetes Australia is grateful to Peter for his honest, open approach to sharing his own experiences, thoughts and feelings about coming to terms with what he agrees, albeit reluctantly, is a disease that won't go away.

There's nothing quite like sharing someone else's journey to help smooth the path for your own. Diabetes Australia commends this book to all people with Type 2 diabetes and is confident that it will be of great value in making that journey, both now and down the track.

Associate Professor *Peter Little*
President
Diabetes Australia

A Word from Nutritionist Catherine Saxelby

You are what you eat

You are what you eat. To put it more colloquially, what you eat today walks and talks tomorrow! I love both these sayings because they so powerfully yet simply tell us the importance of good nutrition.

Rising rates of obesity and sedentary lives are fuelling an 'epidemic' of diabetes. As more and more Australians are diagnosed with Type 2 diabetes, the call for a healthier way of eating is urgent.

Much has been written about what we should or shouldn't eat over the past few years. From the no-carb approach of the Atkins Diet to the ever-expanding research into the Glycaemic Index (GI), it's hard not to be confused about what to put on your plate. Nevertheless, the essentials of healthy eating don't change whether you have a dietary problem or just want to eat for energy and health.

Having diabetes doesn't mean a special diet that's different from everyone else's. The ideal diet for diabetes is much the same as a healthy diet for all of us: low in saturated fat, high in fibre, moderate in salt, added sugar and refined starches, and would use carbohydrates that are wholegrain or low GI. It should incorporate a wide variety of fruit, vegetables, nuts, legumes, lean meats, fish, low-fat dairy foods and 'good' fat—all those basic, healthy staples that our grandparents would have told us to eat.

We should also aim to eat less 'junk'—you all know what I mean—less refined and processed foods. We don't want to eliminate all convenience products but we're clearly consuming too many of those 'instant' dinner, 'just microwave' meals and take-aways.

Anyone with diabetes is advised to:
- Eat regular meals spread evenly over the day. Don't skip meals.
- Eat plenty of vegetables, salads and fruit. The official recommendation is to eat '2+5', which translates to two servings of fruit plus five servings of vegetables each day. Eat more if you want to.
- Choose foods low in saturated fat.
- Use less fat and make sure any fat you eat is a healthy fat.
- Choose 'better' carbohydrates that are wholegrain and low GI.
- Make exercise a priority and do it regularly.
- Lose excess weight if you need to.

How Peter does it

In this book, Peter Howard shows how to create diabetes-friendly dishes that fit with these suggestions.

Starting with healthy basic ingredients, he makes everything look and taste wonderful—without frying or rich sauces, cooking without heaps of butter or cream and he includes plenty of those all-important vegetables and salads.

Congratulations to Peter on creating such light, fresh and interesting recipes to inspire and motivate us. It would not have been easy for Peter, with his background in the culinary arts and always tempted by yet another invitation to sample a new gourmet product or taste some fine wine.

If Peter can do it, so can you!

Catherine Saxelby
BSc, Grad Dip Nutrition and Dietetics (Syd), APD,
AIFST
Dietitian and author of *Nutrition for Life*

Introduction

'Nothing succeeds like excess' was my mantra for many years and boy did I live it. My job as a food editor on national television for many years opened the doors to so many opportunities to be as bad as I liked and to eat and drink as much as I liked. It was the perfect excuse: 'This is what I do for a living'; so I threw my self into my job with a passion and gusto that few could believe.

My long-suffering and wonderful doctor for many years, Dr Don Wilton, kept telling me to adjust or mend my Bacchanalian ways or accept the dreaded results. In my mind that was always going to be someone else ... never me.

All that changed when my current doctor, Andrew McNaught, let me have the 'good' news on 23 December, 2004 that I have Type 2 diabetes and now was the time to adjust or cop the consequences—which I can tell you he outlined without any gloss or lies. Adjust and live or keep on and ... the rest you can imagine, especially if you are either a diabetic or involved with someone who is.

This book is written for people who suffer with Type 2 diabetes and is written by someone who has the disease. Even now, after months of living with it, I still find it hard to write the word 'disease' because I want to ignore it or want it to go away. I know, like so many folk now, that we have a disease that will not go away but can be controlled by diet, exercise (at least 30 minutes to an hour everyday) and restraint or discipline. I know many diabetics before me have faced and won this same dilemma. I'm sure, for each of us, it is a very difficult private battle. We have to forgive ourselves for arriving at this stage and just get on with life ... and our newfound lifestyle.

I decided to write my eating experiences to share with so many people who have supported me for years with my other cookbooks and multiple media and personal appearances. When I started to investigate what we could eat, I did contemplate thc alternative to looking after myself. I do have so much to live for and a really good life, so the alternative had to be dismissed. However, that still did not appease the thought of no more fats—at least to the degree that I used to ingest anyway. What would I do without the cream on my puddings? How could I live on only two standard glasses of red wine a day—and have two dry days a week as well? How was I going to do this—and lose weight too?

Like so many of us, I had to find the determination to do this. Lose weight, exercise, watch what I drink—essentially change my lifestyle completely or perish. That was the hard bit to acknowledge—the perish bit. Did you notice that when you begin to lose weight, you find an amazing amount of energy? Your blood pressure drops? And your blood sugar levels sort themselves out?

What has developing Type 2 diabetes meant to

me? I see it as a real wake-up call and it has strengthened my resolve to become healthy.

I have set to paper the recipes that I live by and adhere to 99 per cent of the time. Because this change in our lives is for the long haul, we want wonderful flavoursome, tasty dishes that all diabetics can enjoy. This makes the transition easy. More importantly, these scrumptious dishes make it easier for us to stick with it, because it is for the rest of our lives.

It is, of course, important to limit the overall quantity of food eaten and to follow the suggested serving sizes in the recipes. People with diabetes must take into account other foods in the diet. You do not need to eat an entree, main and desert at every meal, even if they are healthy. Keep track of your total carbohydrate intake, as some of my snacks are a touch high in carbo.

My intake of fruit has certainly improved, as has my fibre intake. I am now surprising people by how well I look—even myself. It almost sounds as though I am happy to be a diabetic. I am not over-joyed but know that I have a disease that I can treat with exercise, diet control and by watching my alcoholic drinking habits. I also know that there is so much great tasting, wholesome, nutritious food around that I can eat with excitement and satisfaction.

Modern eating habits, with so much refined and pre-prepared fast food, mean we hand over the responsibility to others to feed us. Do we really know what goes into most of our foods and do we care? The reality is that we folk with diabetes (and everyone really) have to care. It is crucial you read the nutritional bar/breakdowns on prepared food you buy. Do you have enough time to cook for yourself? Of course you do and—if you examine the excuses you've made—you'll find it's because you've fooled yourself into believing you don't. Perhaps more to the point, you have to make the time to look after your dietary requirements now.

There is so much information available from the various Diabetes Australia organisations. Their nutritional information is fantastic and I have been aided enormously by Alan Barclay, the research and development manager of Diabetes Australia NSW and his colleague, Carole Webster, the national publications manager for Diabetes Australia. My thanks also to the President of Diabetes Australia, Professor Peter Little for his kind words.

The cold, hard fact we folk with Type 2 diabetes have to understand is that we *must* find the time to cook and prepare totally good food and love it. The way food is packaged currently means you can do this and more to take your life into your hands and accept the responsibility of living and loving yourself. It is a very good way to live your life—your new healthy lifestyle.

Peter Howard

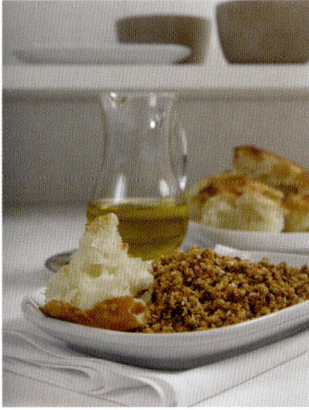

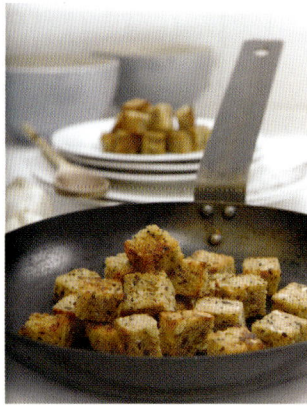

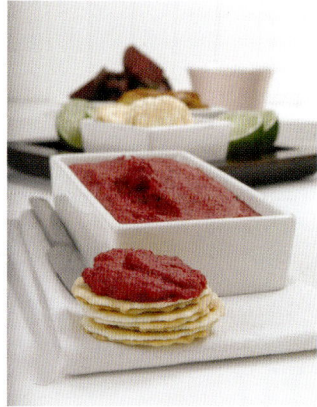

BASICS

I always end up with a group of recipes from each book I write that I think should be there all the time—and they seem basic.

The recipes in this section can be used in whatever application you want and they will become standards for you to have on hand forever.

Beetroot Pinto Bean Hummus

Preparation time: 10 minutes
Makes: 3–4 cups

2 cups cooked pinto beans
200g cooked beetroot, chopped
2 tablespoons lime juice
2 tablespoons organic tahini
1 teaspoon white sesame seeds
½ teaspoon ground white pepper
1 teaspoon cumin, powdered
¼ cup evaporated milk (98.5% fat-free)

Puree all ingredients to a rough paste in a processor or with a hand blender. Store in an airtight container in the refrigerator for up to 7 days.

I use this instead of butter or spread. It is delicious and you only need a small amount. You can substitute other beans for pinto beans, but I find them so easy to use and versatile.

Nutritional information: amounts per serve standard serve size: 29g	
Energy (kJ)	150
Protein (g)	1.8
Total Fat (g)	1.5
Saturated Fat (g)	0.2
Total Carbohydrate (g)	3
Sugars (g)	1.3
Fibre (g)	1.4
Sodium (mg)	54
G.I.	low

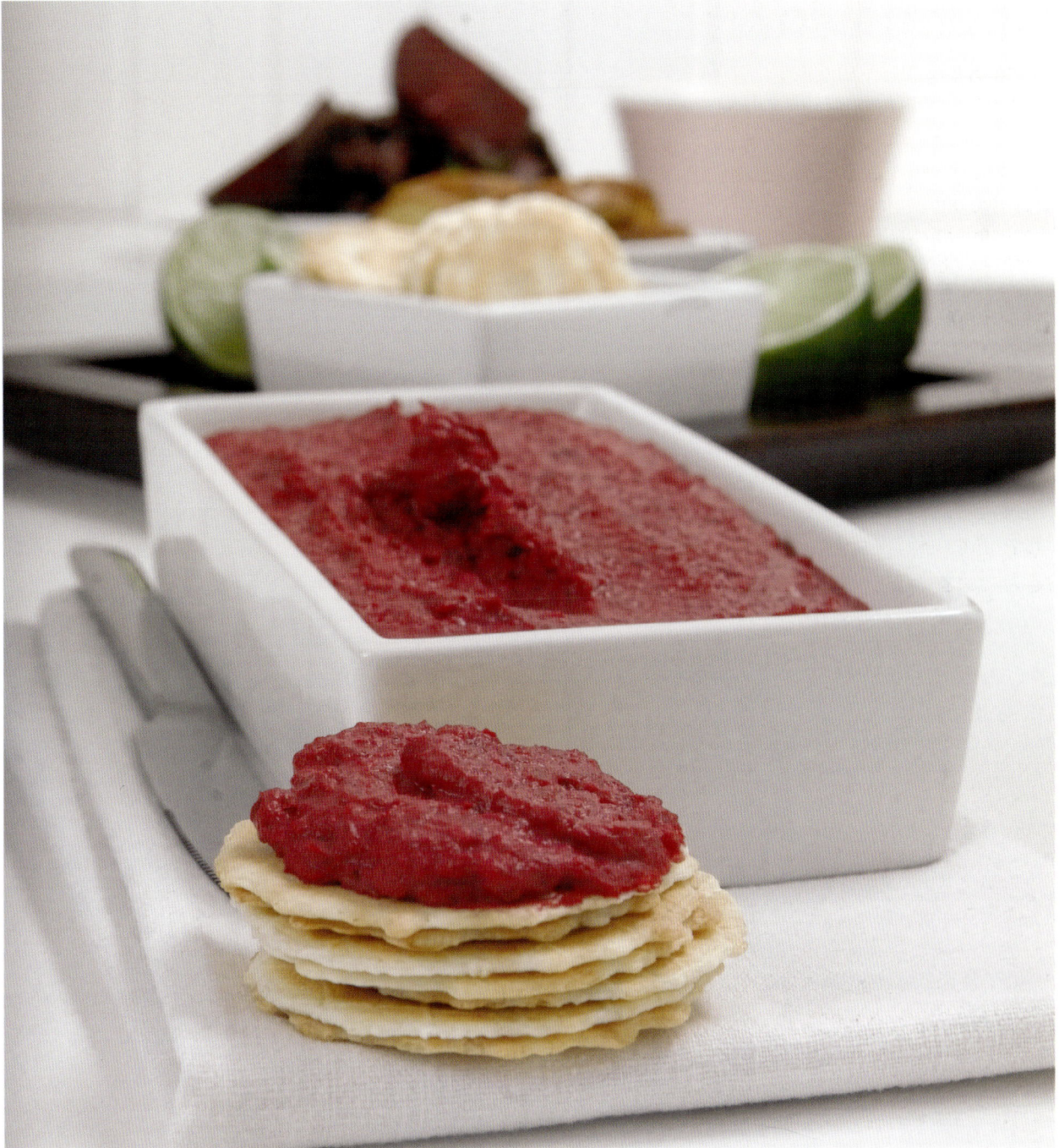

Chermoula

Preparation time: 5 minutes
Makes: 1–2 cups

1 medium onion, very finely chopped/minced
2 teaspoons coriander leaves, finely chopped
4 teaspoons parsley, finely chopped
2 cloves garlic, minced
4 teaspoons cumin seeds, ground
2 teaspoons mild paprika
1 teaspoon powdered turmeric
¼ teaspoon cayenne pepper
¼ teaspoon each of salt and ground black pepper.

Nutritional information: amounts for whole recipe	
Energy (kJ)	175
Protein (g)	2
Total Fat (g)	0.3
Saturated Fat (g)	0.05
Total Carbohydrate (g)	6
Sugars (g)	4
Fibre (g)	3
Sodium (mg)	620
G.I.	n/a

Mix all the ingredients together and use as required to flavour meats.

This versatile sprinkle or rub is a Moroccan delight that is delicious on fish, lamb and chicken. It will store in the refrigerator for up 7 days in an airtight container.

Olive Parsley Paste

Preparation time: 10 minutes
Makes: 1–2 cups

80g green olives, seeds removed
1 cup loosely packed curly parsley
1 tablespoon fresh oregano, chopped
2 lemons, grated zest only
juice of one of the lemons
3 cloves garlic, peeled and roughly chopped
1 tablespoon hazelnuts, skins on and roughly chopped

Nutritional information: amounts for whole recipe	
Energy (kJ)	110
Protein (g)	0.6
Total Fat (g)	1.2
Saturated Fat (g)	0.1
Total Carbohydrate (g)	3
Sugars (g)	2.5
Fibre (g)	1.1
Sodium (mg)	70
G.I.	n/a

Put all ingredients into a processor and work to a rough paste. Will store in the refrigerator for up to seven days in an airtight container. Rub on meat and vegetables, before or after roasting, for added zest.

Chickpea Hummus

Preparation time: 5 minutes
Makes: 2 cups

350g cooked chickpeas
2 cloves garlic, roughly chopped
3 tablespoons lemon juice
2 tablespoons tahini
1 teaspoon white sesame seeds
½ teaspoon ground white pepper
1 teaspoon powdered cumin
3 tablespoons natural no-fat yoghurt
1 tablespoon water

Puree all ingredients to a rough paste in a processor or with a hand blender. Store, refrigerated, in an airtight container for up to seven days.

If you're a hummus aficionado, you will notice a difference in the texture, as it is usually made with a generous quantity of olive oil. It is normally stored under olive oil, which is mixed in as you eat it. I have resisted the oil and this is a very good snack base that I with vegetable sticks around mid-afternoon, when I am peckish.

I have used both the canned and dry chickpeas for this recipe—both work well. Interestingly, a 375g packet of dried peas—soaked for 4 hours—will cook (by boiling in fresh water) in around 45 minutes and yield 850g of cooked peas. I use the leftover peas in a quick chilli or curry dish.

Nutritional information: amounts for whole recipe	
Energy (kJ)	2810
Protein (g)	32
Total Fat (g)	33
Saturated Fat (g)	4.2
Total Carbohydrate (g)	51
Sugars (g)	4.5
Fibre (g)	23
Sodium (mg)	910
G.I.	low

Garlic Croutons

Preparation time: 5 minutes
Cooking time: 10 minutes
Makes: 4 serves

4 slices day old rye and linseed bread or similar (I use Burgen)
1 tablespoon garlic, crushed
spray canola oil

1. Cut the bread into 2cm squares. Place into a non-stick frying pan, add the garlic and spray with oil. Put on a medium heat and toss to colour and crisp. You need to keep the croutons moving so the garlic doesn't discolour.
2. Tip onto a kitchen towelling-lined plate and cool. Use when ready.

These are flavour bombs with that added crunch for salad and soups. They store well in an airtight container and you'll be surprised where you will find a use for them. You will use them all at once for 4 serves. If you make them a little bigger, you can use them as a small biscuit for dips.

Nutritional information: amounts per serve	
Energy (kJ)	440
Protein (g)	4
Total Fat (g)	2.5
Saturated Fat (g)	0.5
Total Carbohydrate (g)	15
Sugars (g)	1
Fibre (g)	3
Sodium (mg)	180
G.I.	low

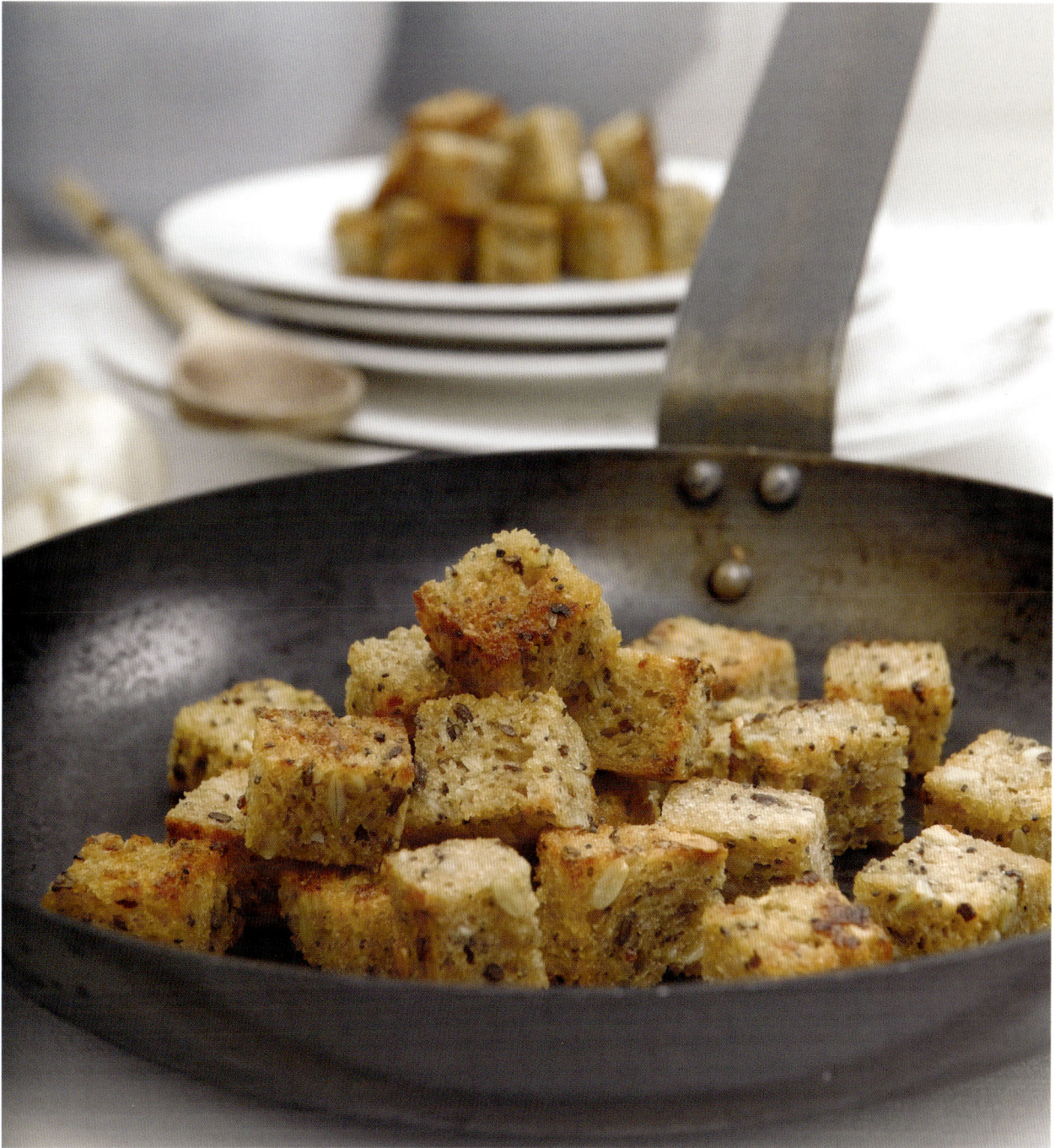

My Dukkah

Preparation time: 10 minutes
Cooking time: 5 minutes
Makes: 1½ cups

100 almonds, skin on
60g pine nuts
20g linseeds
1 teaspoon ground coriander
1 teaspoon ground cumin
1 teaspoon white sesame seeds
½ teaspoon chilli powder
1 teaspoon Szechuan peppercorns

1. Dry roast the almonds, pine nuts and linseeds over medium heat. Cool and tip into a food processor. Dry roasting is where the nuts and seeds are pan-fried dry without any added moisture or fat. This helps to bring out flavours and natural oils.
2. Add the coriander, cumin, sesame seeds, chilli and Szechuan pepper. Work to a rough granular mixture—not a paste. Store in an airtight container.

I use this constantly because of the great flavour and texture. You can use it with chicken for pan-frying, on lamb before and during barbecuing or sprinkle it over salads. As a snack dip a good bread to into a small amount of olive oil and then dip that into the dukkah mix.

The linseeds are very nutritious and have an oil that comes out very quickly when heated. Do watch the pine nuts and the linseeds when dry roasting them as they both burn very quickly.

Nutritional information: amounts per whole recipe	
Energy (kJ)	6000
Protein (g)	37
Total Fat (g)	120
Saturated Fat (g)	8
Total Carbohydrate (g)	9
Sugars (g)	9
Fibre (g)	8
Sodium (mg)	25
G.I.	n/a

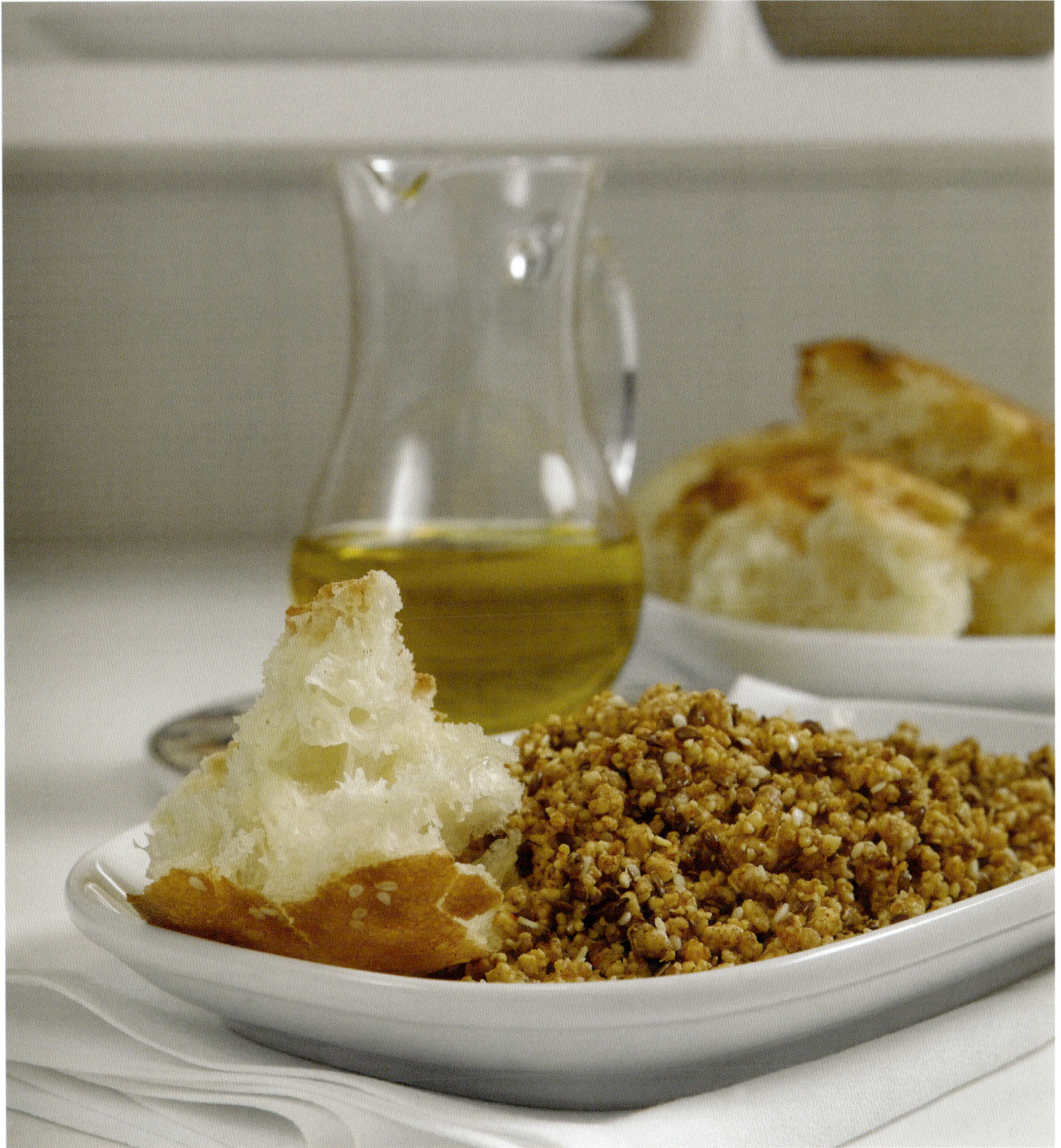

Olive Oil Pastry

Preparation time: 15 minutes

1½ cups organic plain flour (or good plain flour)
60 ml (¼ cup) olive oil (I use extra virgin olive oil)
1 egg yolk
3–3½ tablespoons very cold water

1. Put the flour, oil and egg yolk into a food processor bowl. Process until the mixture resembles breadcrumbs.
2. Pour in 3 tablespoons of water with machine working. Stop the motor when the mixture starts to ball around the cutter. You may need to add more water depending on the mix.
3. Tip out onto a lightly floured bench and work into a dough.

You can use this pastry for various savoury needs—or sweet needs for that matter.

This pastry can be rolled out and fitted into flan or pie tins before being put into the freezer for 45 minutes. Remove and blind bake.

Nutritional information: amounts for whole recipe	
Energy (kJ)	5360
Protein (g)	25
Total Fat (g)	62
Saturated Fat (g)	9.5
Total Carbohydrate (g)	151
Sugars (g)	0.5
Fibre (g)	8
Sodium (mg)	71
G.I.	

To blind bake:

Place baking paper over the pastry and fill with rice, dried beans or pastry weights.

Bake in 180°C oven (fan-forced 160°C) for 10 minutes then remove paper and rice/beans/weights. Bake for another 10 minutes.

Sri Lankan Curry Powder

Preparation time: 20 minutes
Cooking time: 5 minutes
Makes: 1–2 cups

3 tablespoons coriander seeds
1½ tablespoons cumin seeds
1 teaspoon fennel seeds
1 teaspoon basmati rice
10–15 curry leaves
10 fenugreek seeds
2 small dried red chillies
3 whole cloves
1 x 8cm cinnamon stick
4 cardamom pods
2 large garlic cloves, roughly sliced

1. Dry roast the coriander, cumin and fennel seeds in a non-stick pan until lightly browned. Tip out to cool. Dry roast the rice until lightly browned. Tip out to cool.
2. In a non-stick pan, dry roast the curry leaves, fenugreek, chillies, cloves, cinnamon, cardamom and garlic for a few minutes. Cool and combine with the other ingredients.
3. Grind in a mortar and pestle or in a small food processor to a powder. Store in an airtight container.

You may wonder why all the ingredients are not dry roasted together. This is because the first three—the coriander, cumin and fennel—colour very quickly. I use dry pre-roasted garlic for convenience in this exotic and genuine curry powder—from the hands of Chef Peter Kuravita and generations of his relatives.

Nutritional information: amounts for whole recipe	
Energy (kJ)	1760
Protein (g)	16.5
Total Fat (g)	34
Saturated Fat (g)	4
Total Carbohydrate (g)	9
Sugars (g)	2
Fibre (g)	9
Sodium (mg)	11
G.I.	n/a

Buckwheat Crepes

Makes: 8 crepes

¾ cup buckwheat flour
1 large egg
1 cup 98% fat-free milk
spray oil (canola or olive)

1. Beat the flour with the egg and milk and let sit for 30 minutes before use.
2. To make the pancakes, spray a minute amount of oil onto a non-stick crepe pan or a pan you use for crepes/pancakes. Using a ladle, pour in enough batter to make the size you want—around 18 cm in diameter. When small bubbles start to appear, flip over and repeat until all batter is used.
3. These cool quickly so keep warm on a low heat in the oven if required.

Nutritional information: amounts per crepe	
Energy (kJ)	370
Protein (g)	4
Total Fat (g)	2
Saturated Fat (g)	0.5
Total Carbohydrate (g)	13
Sugars (g)	2
Fibre (g)	2
Sodium (mg)	25
G.I.	low

BREAKFAST

It's been called the most important meal of the day and it really is so essential to get off to a good start. Besides the recipes I have in this section, I always have some fresh fruit. I love prunes in my cereal and often munch on them during my morning preparation for breakfast. I always look to see what my day holds. With my busy schedule I may be travelling, having a lunch in a restaurant or eating on the run. I now know how to eat healthily in the hotel breakfast dining areas and know my way around a buffet. My daily routine determines my eating for the day.

I remember that old saying: 'Eat like a king for breakfast, eat like a prince for lunch and eat like a pauper for dinner!'

I try to do this as much as I can. I always start my day with a full tummy!

Asparagus and Salmon Flat Omelette

Preparation and cooking time: 25 minutes
Serves: 4

½ cup cooked asparagus, diced
200g canned red salmon, flaked and drained
¼ cup chives, chopped
1 tablespoon low-fat natural yoghurt
2 medium-sized eggs
4 egg whites
½ teaspoon ground black pepper
½ teaspoon ground allspice
spray canola oil

1. Mix the asparagus, salmon and chives together.
2. Beat the yoghurt, eggs, egg whites, pepper and ground allspice and mix well.
3. Lightly spray a non-stick frying pan and heat to medium. Pour in the egg mixture and stir with a plastic spatula to stop sticking. When it starts to set, stir in the asparagus mixture and cook to continue the setting of the eggs.
4. When the bottom of the omelette is set, put under a very hot grill to lightly brown and finish setting.
5. Serve equal quantities with wholegrain toast.

I use a 20-cm diameter pan (4–5 cm deep). I can turn the omelette out instead of cutting it in the pan, which protects the pan and gives good presentation.

Nutritional information: amounts per serve	
Energy (kJ)	690
Protein (g)	19
Total Fat (g)	9
Saturated Fat (g)	2.5
Total Carbohydrate (g)	1
Sugars (g)	1
Fibre (g)	0.5
Sodium (mg)	415
G.I.	n/a

Mixed Fruit Smoothie

Preparation time: 10 minutes
Serves: 4

300 ml (1¼ cups) skim or fat-reduced milk
200 ml (¾ cup) apple juice
200 ml (¾ cup) fruit salad low-fat yoghurt
1 cup frozen mixed berries
½ cup apple, chopped (skin on)
200g banana, chopped
1 tablespoon psyllium husks
freshly grated nutmeg

1. Put all ingredients, except for the nutmeg, into a blender and combine.
2. Pour into serving glasses and sprinkle with nutmeg.

A great way to start the day, and I often have one of these as a midmorning snack when I am working in the office. Smoothies are quick to prepare and filling.

Nutritional information: amounts per serve	
Energy (kJ)	665
Protein (g)	7.5
Total Fat (g)	0.5
Saturated Fat (g)	0.1
Total Carbohydrate (g)	30
Sugars (g)	28
Fibre (g)	3
Sodium (mg)	75
G.I.	

Grilled Banana On Jam Toast

Preparation time: 5 minutes
Cooking time: 10 minutes
Serves: 4

4 slices rye or soy and linseed bread
4 teaspoons spreadable fruit (no-cane-sugar-added spread)
2 large, ripe Cavendish bananas
4 tablespoons no-fat/low-fat fruit yoghurt

1. Brown the toast on one side.
2. Spoon the spread evenly over the non-browned side of the toast.
3. Top with banana slices or mash the banana onto the spread side of each piece of bread.
4. Grill the bananas until they are lightly browned.
5. Serve topped with a tablespoon of your favourite no-fat or low-fat yoghurt

You may have guessed that I have a sweet tooth from this recipe. You can imagine how I fell on these no-cane-sugar-added fruit spreads, which come in many flavours.

Nutritional information: amounts per serve	
Energy (kJ)	780
Protein (g)	6
Total Fat (g)	2
Saturated Fat (g)	0.3
Total Carbohydrate (g)	35
Sugars (g)	18
Fibre (g)	4
Sodium (mg)	190
G.I.	low

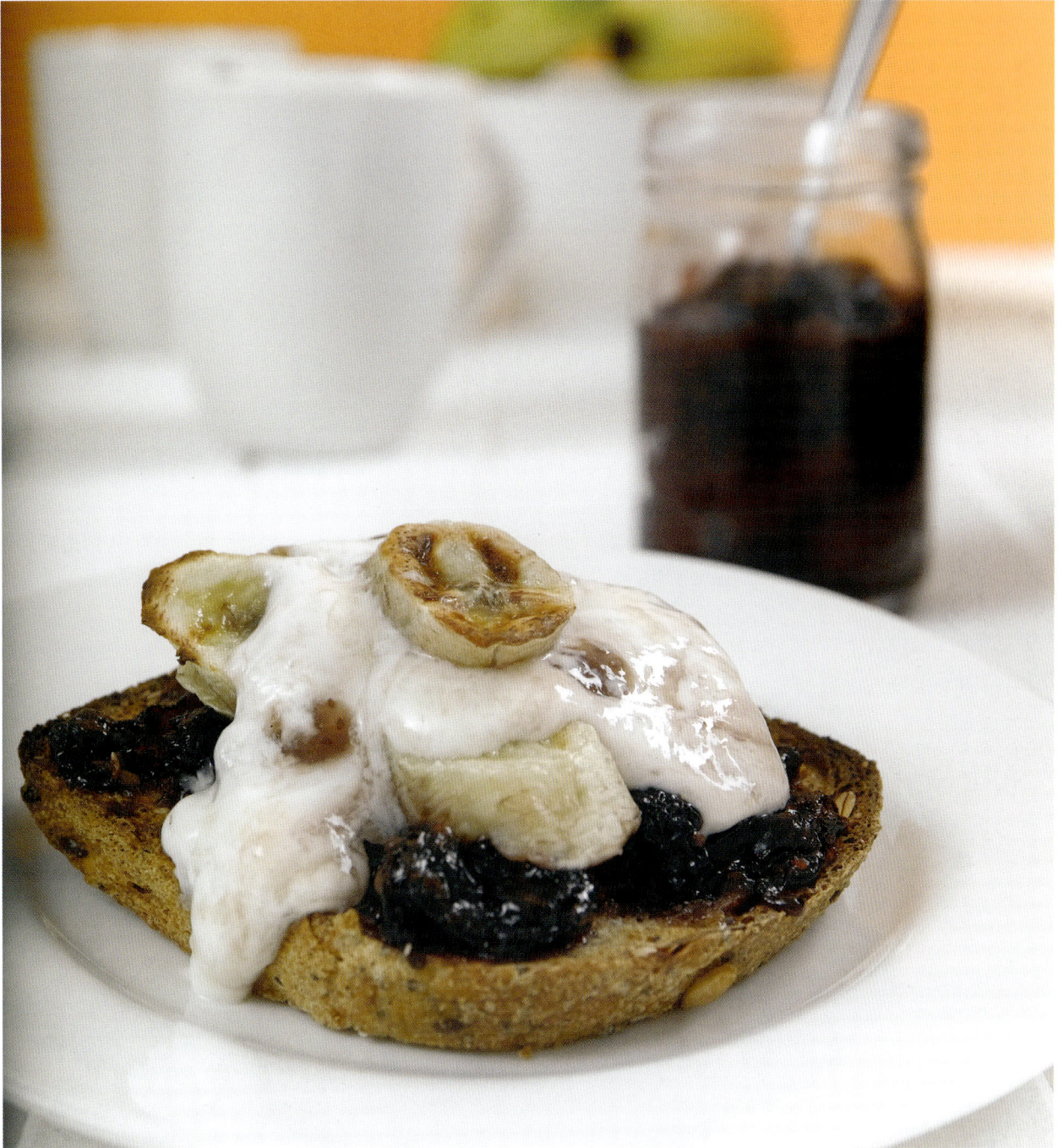

Oven Baked Eggs 'n' Beans

Preparation time: 5 minutes
Cooking time: 25 minutes
Serves: 4

400g low sodium baked beans
4 x 70g eggs at room temperature
2 tablespoons chives, chopped
spray canola oil
8 slices wholemeal, soy and linseed or rye bread

1. Preheat oven 200°C (fan-forced 180°C). Spray four, small ovenproof containers with a smear of oil. I use Chinese dipping bowls.
2. Divide the beans evenly into the four bowls. Break an egg into each one. Place all bowls onto a baking tray and slip into the oven and cook for 25 minutes or until set to your liking. This timing will give you runny egg yolks.
3. Toast the bread. Serve the eggs and beans sprinkled with chives and toast on the side. Add ground black pepper if you like.

These can also be done in the microwave. Cover each bowl with cling wrap, cook them on 70 per cent for 3–4 minutes. I did mine individually as I have a small microwave, but you may be able to do more in a larger oven.

Nutritional information: amounts per serve	
Energy (kJ)	1530
Protein (g)	21
Total Fat (g)	10.5
Saturated Fat (g)	2.5
Total Carbohydrate (g)	42
Sugars (g)	7
Fibre (g)	10
Sodium (mg)	560
G.I.	low

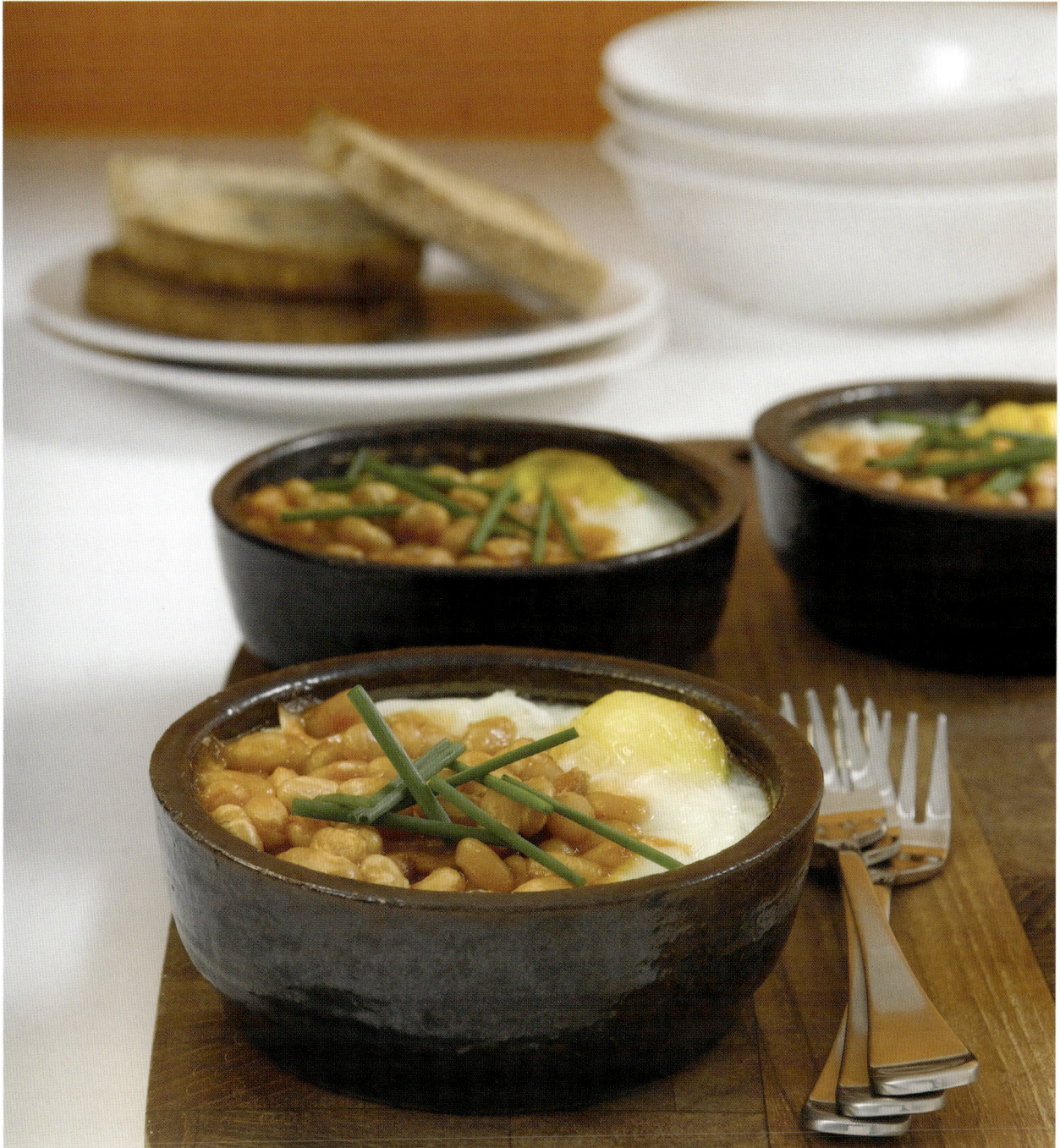

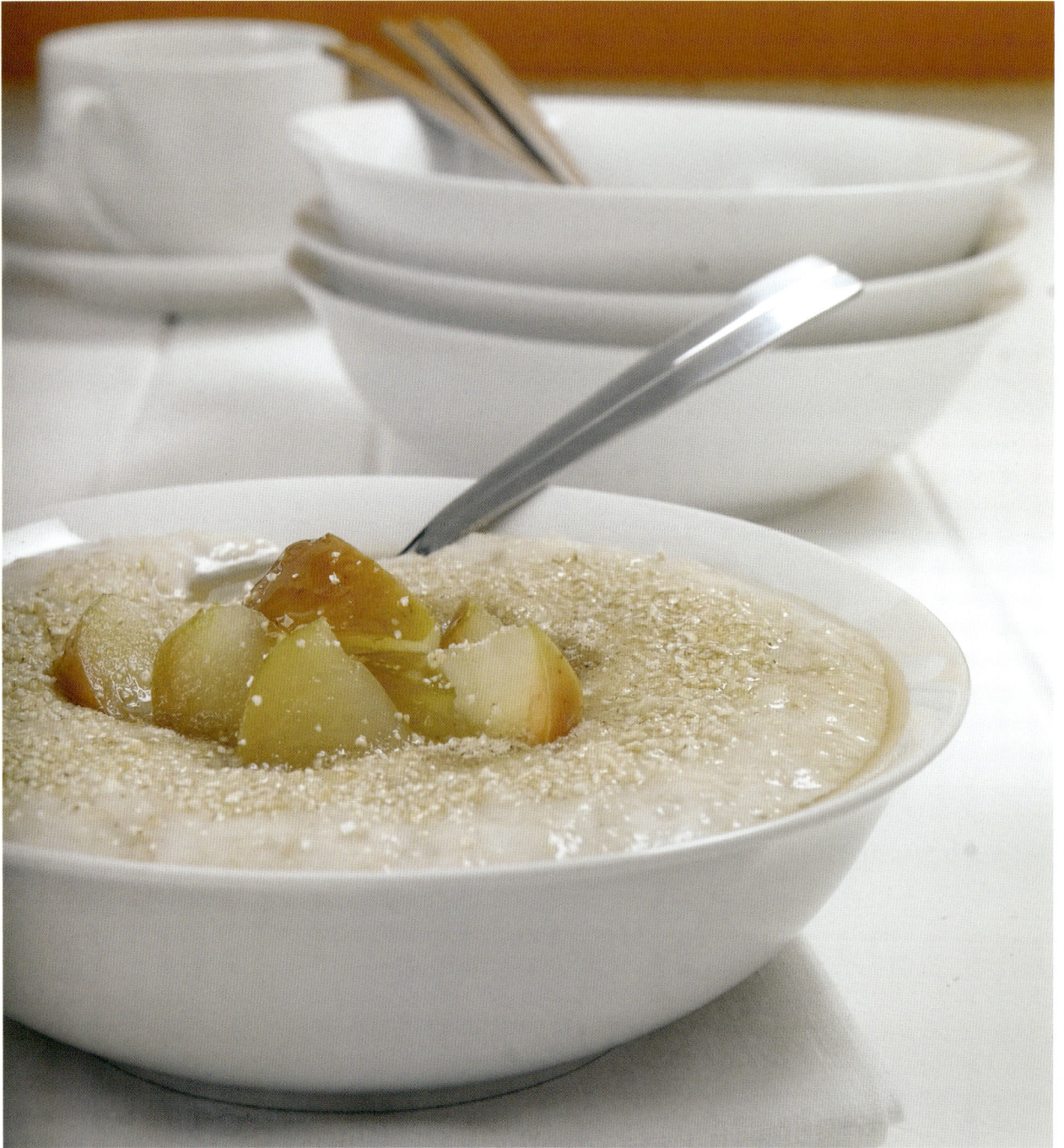

Rolled Oats, Barley Bran and Stewed Ginger Apples

Preparation time: 10 minutes
Cooking time: 10 minutes
Serves: 6

4 medium eating apples (Bonza, Fuji, Burnbrae, etc.)
1 x 4cm-long piece root ginger
2 cups organic or original rolled oats
3 cups water
1 cup skim milk
2 tablespoons psyllium
4 tablespoons barley bran
4 tablespoons honey, preferably organic or yellow box

1. Cut the apples into quarters or eight wedges if larger and remove the core. Put into a saucepan and cover them with water. Slice the ginger finely and add to the apples. Cook at a simmer for 10 minutes. Remove from heat and cool in cooking juices.
2. Cook the oats with the water and milk. Simmer until tender: around 5 minutes.
3. Pour oats out into six individual serving bowls. Top with equal amounts of psyllium, bran, honey and stewed apple to serve.

You can add more milk if you want or even flavoured, non-fat yoghurt.

The apples keep for up to a week if you want to make more than this recipe. The ginger should be washed and scraped, not peeled.

Nutritional information: amounts per serve	
Energy (kJ)	1140
Protein (g)	6
Total Fat (g)	3
Saturated Fat (g)	0.5
Total Carbohydrate (g)	55
Sugars (g)	31
Fibre (g)	5
Sodium (mg)	26
G.I.	low

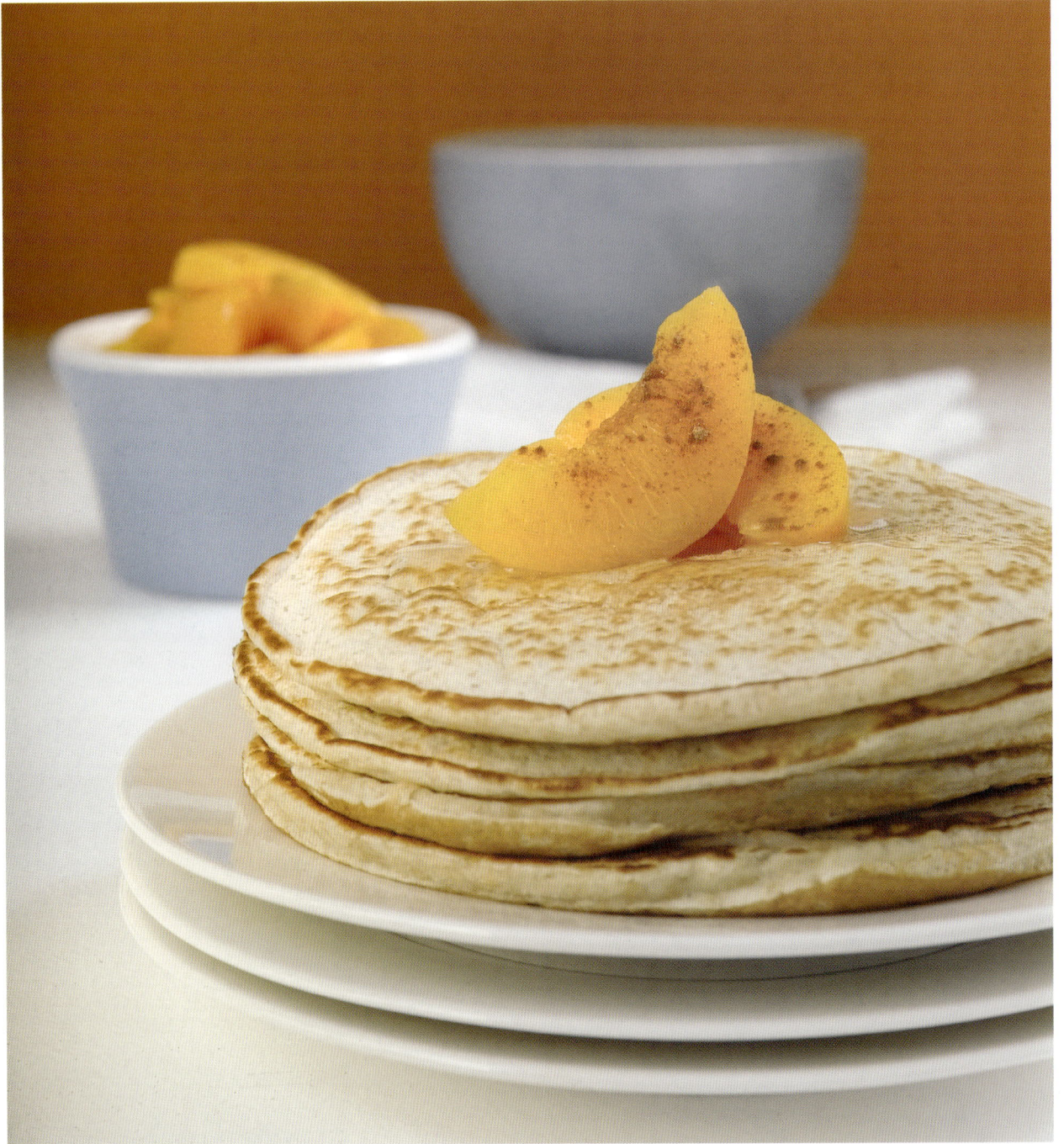

Wholemeal Pancakes and Cinnamon Peaches

Preparation time: 10 minutes
Cooking time: 15 minutes
Makes: 12 pancakes

2 cups wholemeal self-raising flour
2 cups skim milk
1 teaspoon canola oil
1 teaspoon vanilla essence
2 egg whites, beaten until stiff
1 x 410g can sliced peaches, in their own juice
1 teaspoon ground cinnamon
spray canola oil for cooking

1. Mix the flour with milk and oil in a suitable bowl. When combined fold in the egg whites and let sit for 5 minutes.
2. Heat the peaches in their juice with the cinnamon in the microwave until warm.
3. Spray a crepe/pancake pan with minimal oil and cook each pancake. Turn when the bubbles start to appear. Flip over and cook through.
4. Serve the pancakes with peaches and syrup over the top.

These are great served with flavoured non-fat yoghurt and strawberries too. The pancakes can be used for savoury meals too; try them for lunch topped with cold meats and salads; as they stay moist and carry flavour really well.

Nutritional information: amounts per pancake (including peach topping)	
Energy (kJ)	400
Protein (g)	4
Total Fat (g)	1
Saturated Fat (g)	0.1
Total Carbohydrate (g)	16
Sugars (g)	5
Fibre (g)	2.4
Sodium (mg)	140
G.I.	medium

Parsley Pepper Tomato Melt

Preparation time: 5 minutes
Cooking time: 15 minutes
Serves: 4

4 slices rye and linseed bread or similar
2 cups medium-sized tomatoes, diced
¼ cup parsley, chopped
1 tablespoon ground black pepper
1 cup 93% fat-free cheese, grated
½ lemon, juiced

1. Brown the bread on one side.
2. Mix the tomato, parsley and pepper.
3. Place browned bread on tray, toasted side down. Top with the tomato mixture and spread the cheese evenly over each slice. Melt/brown the cheese under griller.
4. Serve sprinkled with the lemon juice.

For a substantial lunch add some mixed lettuce leaves, red onion and tomatoes. Sprinkle the lemon juice over the salad.

Nutritional information: amounts per serve	
Energy (kJ)	770
Protein (g)	15
Total Fat (g)	4
Saturated Fat (g)	2
Total Carbohydrate (g)	18
Sugars (g)	3.5
Fibre (g)	5
Sodium (mg)	380
G.I.	low

LUNCH

This is the meal that perks you up through the middle of the day. I am often glued to the computer or on the run, but I do stop—even just for 10 minutes—and eat good food. A break for lunch is all a part of wellbeing. It rests the brain as well as nourishing the body. The two go together. Eating while walking is not the best way to take in your food. All too often this is what I see.

Another endeavour of mine is to make lunch the main meal of the day. This is not usually possible, but I do try to make dinner a lighter meal. I know I sleep better if I do.

To that end, I have included some hefty, filling dishes for lunch as well as some lighter ones. I have noticed that as I lose weight and eat in a better way, I am not that hungry (read ravenous) all the time or hanging out for dinner.

Lunch, like breakfast, is not a meal to miss. I well remember—in my 'fad' diet days—skipping lunch or having a piece of fruit and trying to make do until dinner. It simply does not work. Now I have lunch and a piece of fruit too.

Almond, Lemon and Peri-Peri Grilled Fillets of Fish

Preparation time: 30 minutes
Cooking time: 5–10 minutes
Serves: 4

4 x 150g fillets white fish (I use Dory fillets)
60g almonds, chopped with the skin on
5 tablespoons 97% fat-free mayonnaise
2 tablespoons lemon juice
1 teaspoon medium Peri-Peri (chilli sauce)
1 teaspoon cumin powder
100g mixed lettuce leaves
 shredded zest and juice of one lemon

1. Trim fillets if needed.
2. Mix the almonds, mayonnaise, lemon juice, Peri-Peri and cumin together. Smear the fish fillets with this mixture and let sit for 20 minutes on a baking tray.
3. Heat the griller to very hot and cook the fish under the griller for 5–10 minutes.
4. Dress the salad leaves with the zest and lemon juice. Use as much of the lemon juice as you like—or as little.
5. Serve the cooked fish with the salad and a carbohydrate, such as hot couscous.

I have always liked spicy foods and it is surprising how well all these ingredients blend together during cooking.

I first saw mayonnaise being used to cook/grill fish in the mid 1990s in Chicago. That was full-oil mayonnaise on salmon—too much fat for that beautiful fish. I have used low-fat mayo for ages now and, with these other ingredients, the mayo takes the place of an oil or other fat.

Take care when lifting the fish to serve. Ensure the topping (the almond mixture) stays on top as it can slide off easily.

Nutritional information: amounts per serve	
Energy (kJ)	940
Protein (g)	31
Total Fat (g)	9
Saturated Fat (g)	1
Total Carbohydrate (g)	4
Sugars (g)	3
Fibre (g)	2
Sodium (mg)	225
G.I.	n/a

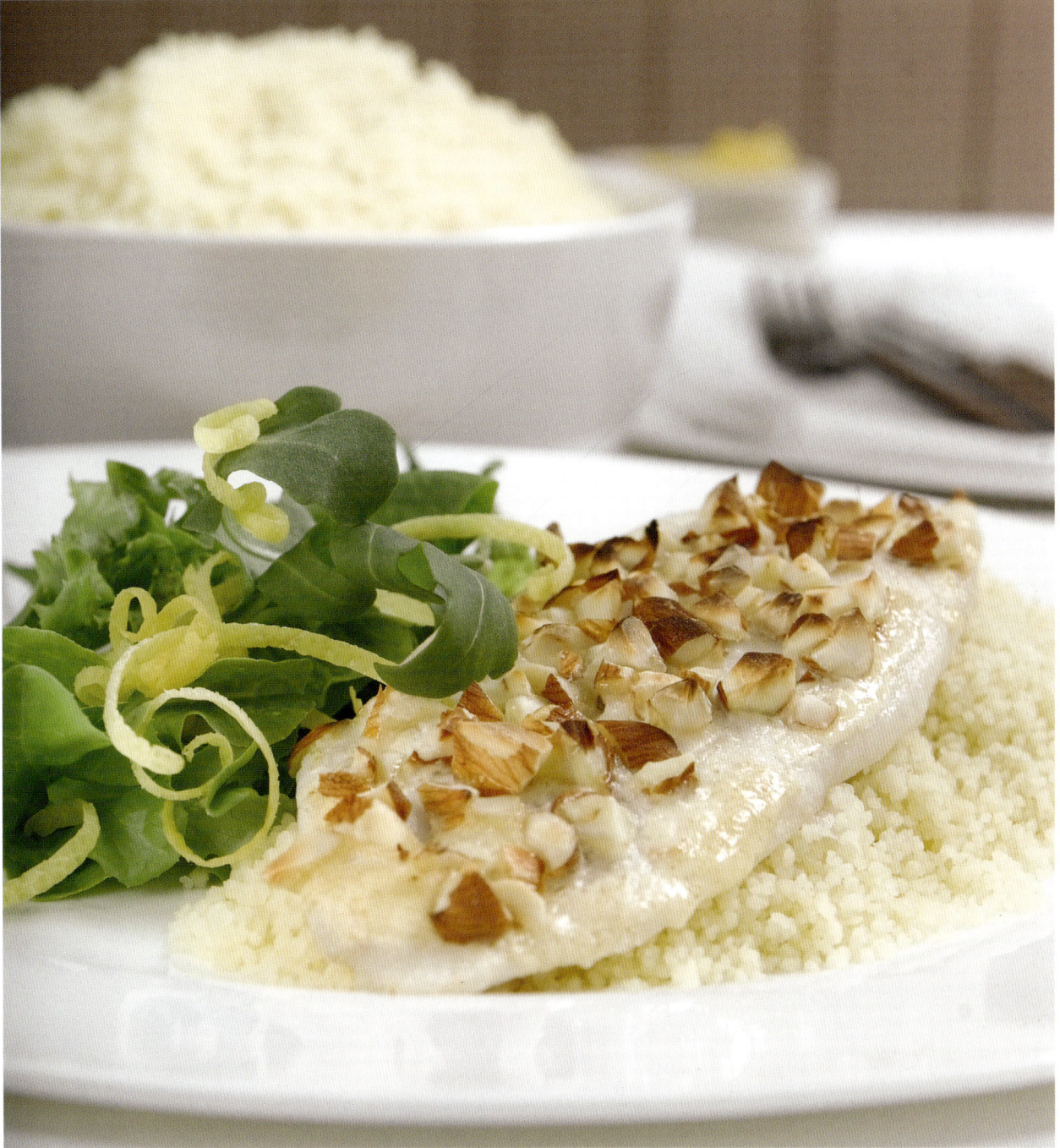

Barbecued Lamb Fajitas

Preparation time: 40 minutes
Cooking time: 5 minutes
Serves: 4

500g mini lamb roasts
1 tablespoon light olive oil
2 tablespoons red wine vinegar
1 teaspoon Mexican spices
1 tablespoon mint, chopped
2 tablespoons dried onion flakes
¼ teaspoon chilli powder (depends on how 'spicy' your powder is)
2 cups lettuce, shredded
1 cup carrot, grated
2 medium salad tomatoes, cut into wedges
½ cup reduced fat/light sour cream
8 wheat flour tortillas

1. Cut the lamb roasts across the grain into 2cm-thick slices, then cut into 1cm-wide strips and place in bowl. Mix the oil, vinegar, Mexican spices, mint, onion flakes and chilli powder together. Pour over the lamb strips and stir to coat the pieces. Cover and refrigerate for at least 30 minutes to 1 hour.
2. Tip the strips onto the hot flat plate on the barbecue. Spread over the plate and cook by tossing and lifting the pieces. Allow them to brown, which will take around 5–6 minutes. Spray the tortillas with oil and heat very quickly on the open char grill.
3. Assemble the fajitas with equal amounts of lettuce, carrot and tomato onto a warmed tortilla. Top with lamb and sour cream. Roll and eat.

I have loved these tasty combinations for years. They are easy and a family favourite. If you can leave the meat to marinade a little longer, they will have a stronger flavour. When you learn how to pronounce them, they are even better. *Far-heat-tars* may be close.

Nutritional information: amounts per serve	
Energy (kJ)	2380
Protein (g)	19
Total Fat (g)	26
Saturated Fat(g)	10
Total Carbohydrate (g)	39
Sugar (g)	6
Fibre (g)	4.5
Sodium (mg)	430
GI	low

Barbecued Snapper Fillets and Vegetables with Citrus Dressing

Preparation time: 15 minutes
Cooking time: 10 minutes
Serves: 4

For the fish

Spray canola oil
4 x 150g snapper fillets
4 large, thick red onion rings,
4 red capsicum cheeks
4 medium-sized zucchinis, trimmed
and halved lengthwise
dill sprigs
ground black pepper

For the dressing

1 tablespoon olive oil
1 teaspoon orange zest, finely grated
1 teaspoon lemon zest, finely grated
1 clove garlic, minced
salt and pepper to taste
⅓ cup lemon juice
⅓ cup orange juice

1. Spray the fish fillets with oil and set to one side. Skewer the onion rings with toothpicks to keep whole, spray the vegetables and cook over medium heat on the barbecue's flat plate.
2. Put the fish on the flat plate, cut side down and cook over medium heat. Spray with a little more oil and turn over to skin side.
3. Make the dressing by whisking the oil into the zests, garlic, salt and pepper. Once combined, whisk in the juices slowly.
4. Assemble the dish by placing the onion rings in the middle of each plate, top with capsicum cheeks and zucchini halves. Top this with fish, spoon over the dressing and decorate with dill sprigs. Serve with cooked basmati rice or a carbohydrate of your choice—not potatoes.

As with any fish, do not overcook it or the fish ends up dry and uninviting. When you turn fish that has skin on it, it is best to place the spatula on top of the cooked side to stop it from curling.

Nutritional information: amounts per serve	
Energy (kJ)	370
Protein (g)	9
Total Fat (g)	2.5
Saturated Fat (g)	0.5
Total Carbohydrate (g)	6.5
Sugars (g)	6
Fibre (g)	2.0
Sodium (mg)	55
G.I.	n/a

Chicken, Celery, Apple and Walnut with Lime Mayo

Preparation time: 10 minutes
Serves: 4

2 cups cooked, skinless white chicken meat, diced
2 cups celery, diced
1 cup apple, diced
½ cup walnuts, roughly broken
1 tablespoon chives, chopped
½ cup low-fat mayonnaise
¼ cup lime juice
ground white pepper to taste

Mix the chicken, celery, apple, walnuts and chives. Stir the mayo, lime and pepper together and pour over the chicken mix. Tumble well and serve immediately over shredded lettuce or mixed leaves.

I always cook my own chicken as I can remove the skin beforehand. Normally I use free range/organic chickens. They have so much rich flavour that I find I need to eat less because that richness is filling. Invariably I poach the chickens in aromatic vegetable-enhanced water for a very short time and let them sit in the water to cool. I use the carcass to make stock because I can then control the salt used.

Nutritional information: amounts for whole recipe	
Energy (kJ)	1375
Protein (g)	21
Total Fat (g)	21
Saturated Fat (g)	2.6
Total Carbohydrate (g)	11.5
Sugars (g)	9
Fibre (g)	3
Sodium (mg)	360
G.I.	low

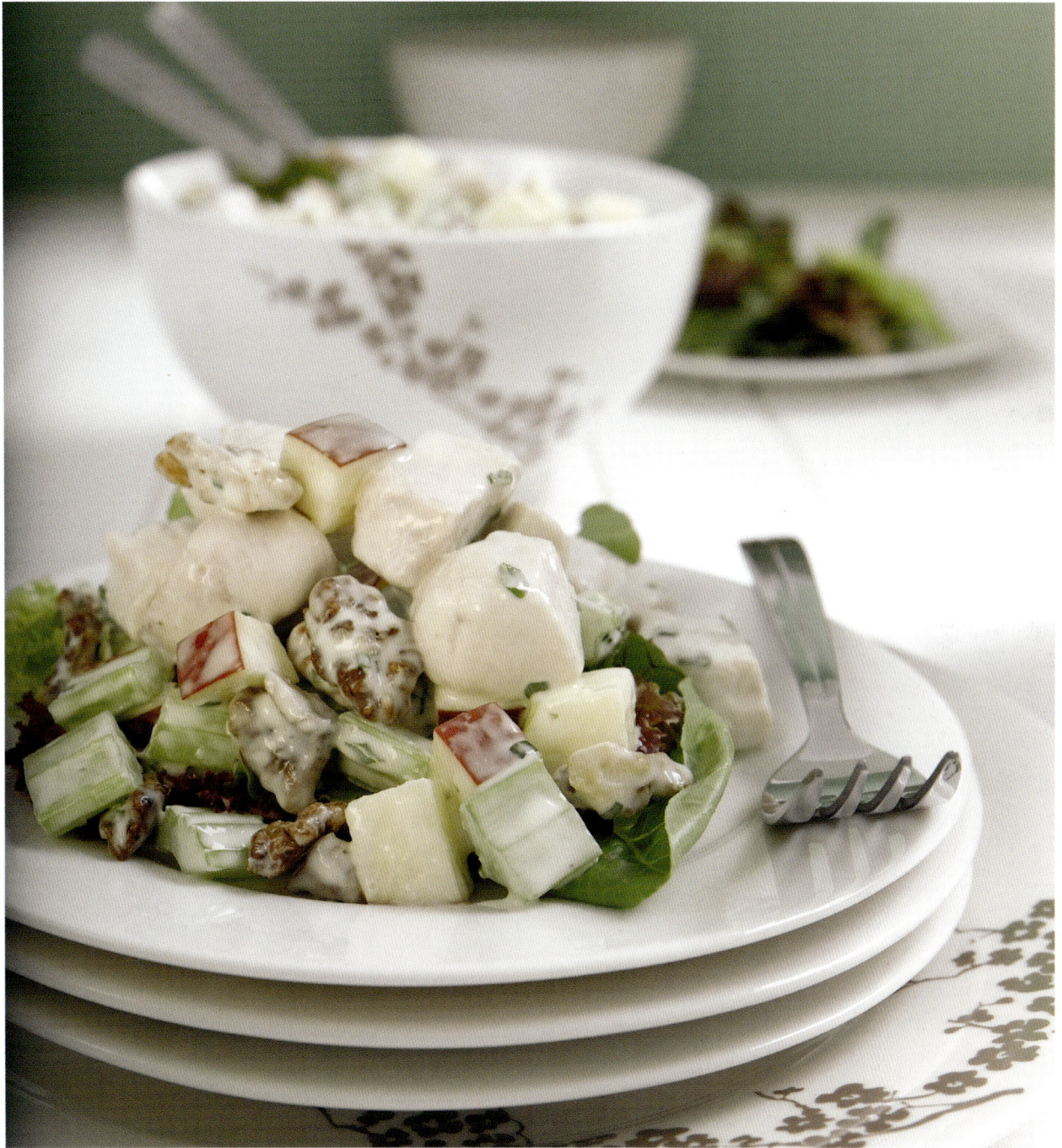

Chicken with Corn and Mango Salsa

Preparation time: 20 minutes
Cooking time: 15 minutes for the chicken
Serves: 4

For the Chicken

400g cooked skinless, boneless chicken breast
100g (1 bag) mixed baby lettuce leaves
20 cooked asparagus tips
1 cup cooked unpeeled potatoes, diced

For the Salsa

1 cup mango flesh, diced
1 cup corn kernels, canned or bottled
1 very small red onion, finely diced
1 small banana chilli, deseeded and minced
1 tablespoon coriander, chopped
salt and ground black pepper to taste
3 tablespoons apple cider vinegar
1 tablespoon mustard seed oil

1. Cut the chicken meat into bite-sized pieces and set to one side.
2. Divide the lettuce leaves onto four plates. Top with equal amounts of asparagus, potatoes and chicken.
3. Make the salsa by combining all ingredients and stirring well. Spoon the salsa over the salad ingredients and serve immediately.

I must confess that I use very little salt anymore and have adjusted to the taste of natural, flavoursome foods. Every now and then I do have a little salt, but it is up to you if you use it or not. My mum hardly ever used salt on our tasty homegrown veggies in my childhood. She maintains that if you don't get used to it as a child you won't ever—some homegrown philosophy.

Nutritional information: amounts per serve	
Energy (kJ)	1350
Protein (g)	30
Total Fat (g)	13
Saturated Fat (g)	3
Total Carbohydrate (g)	17
Sugars (g)	10
Fibre (g)	4
Sodium (mg)	245
G.I.	low

Globe Artichokes and Broad Beans, Tomato Vinaigrette

Preparation time: 20 minutes
Cooking time: 35 minutes
Serves: 4

4 globe artichokes,
1 lemon, halved
cooking string, cut into 4 lengths to tie around
the artichokes
1½ tablespoons extra virgin olive oil
2 tablespoons onion, diced
2 tablespoons lemon juice, from the halves
300g broad beans (fresh or frozen)

For the dressing

1½ tablespoons extra virgin olive oi
2 tablespoons white Balsamic vinegar
½ cup tomato flesh, roughly chopped, peeled
and deseeded
salt flakes and ground black pepper
basil leaves for decoration

1. Trim the artichokes by cutting off a third of the top part. Break away the large, protruding outside leaves. Cut the stem to about 10cm from the base of the artichokes. Tie the string around the artichokes' widest part to keep the shape. Smear the artichokes with the half lemon to retard discolouring.
2. Heat the olive oil in a saucepan and cook the onions for a minute, lift from the heat to cool and pack the prepared artichokes into the saucepan. Add the lemon juice and beans and top with water. Cover and simmer for 30 minutes.
3. Remove from heat, cool a little and lift artichokes carefully from the water (keep warm). Remove the beans and, when cool enough, peel if you like.
4. Whisk the oil until it is slightly aerated. Continue whisking as you add the vinegar. Stir in tomato flesh and season with salt and pepper.
5. Remove the string from the artichokes and place into the centre of plates. Spoon over some broad beans, spoon the tomato vinaigrette around the base and rip the basil leaves to scatter around the artichokes.

Nutritional information: amounts per serve	
Energy (kJ)	790
Protein (g)	11
Total Fat (g)	10
Saturated Fat (g)	1.3
Total Carbohydrate (g)	9
Sugars (g)	3
Fibre (g)	6
Sodium (mg)	315
G.I.	n/a

Kumara and Ricotta Layered Stack

Preparation time: 5–10 minutes
Cooking: 10 minutes
Makes: 4 serves

2 cups kumara (orange sweet potato) pieces, around 2cm square
2 tablespoons mustard seed oil or vegetable oil
1 teaspoon caraway seeds
300g reduced fat ricotta
100g low-fat natural yoghurt
1 tablespoon curry powder
4 whole slices mountain bread (98% fat-free)
150g semi-roasted tomatoes, roughly chopped
mixed salad leaves
lemon juice
ground black pepper

1. Pre-heat oven to 200ºC (fan-forced 180ºC)
2. Rub the kumara with oil and brown in oven. Remove, sprinkle with caraway seeds and let cool.
3. Mix the ricotta, yoghurt and curry powder well.
4. Line a baking tray with baking paper. Spread each piece of bread with ricotta mix. Put one in the bottom of the tray. Layer the ingredients in this order: kumara, bread slice, tomatoes, bread slice, kumara and top with last bread slice inverted to give clean top to the stack. Lightly press, cover with cling wrap and refrigerate for 1 hour.
5. To serve, invert the stack onto a cutting board; cut in half to form two smaller rectangles or cut into quarters. Serve on individual plates with lemon doused salad leaves and sprinkle with ground black pepper.

This is the first recipe I wrote for this book. It is one of my favourites and I serve it as a light lunch meal. Friends who have tasted it comment on was how tasty it is—if only they realised how healthy it is too.

Nutritional information: amounts per serve	
Energy (kJ)	1340
Protein (g)	14
Total Fat (g)	17
Saturated Fat (g)	5.5
Total Carbohydrate (g)	27
Sugars (g)	9
Fibre (g)	4
Sodium (mg)	290
G.I.	low

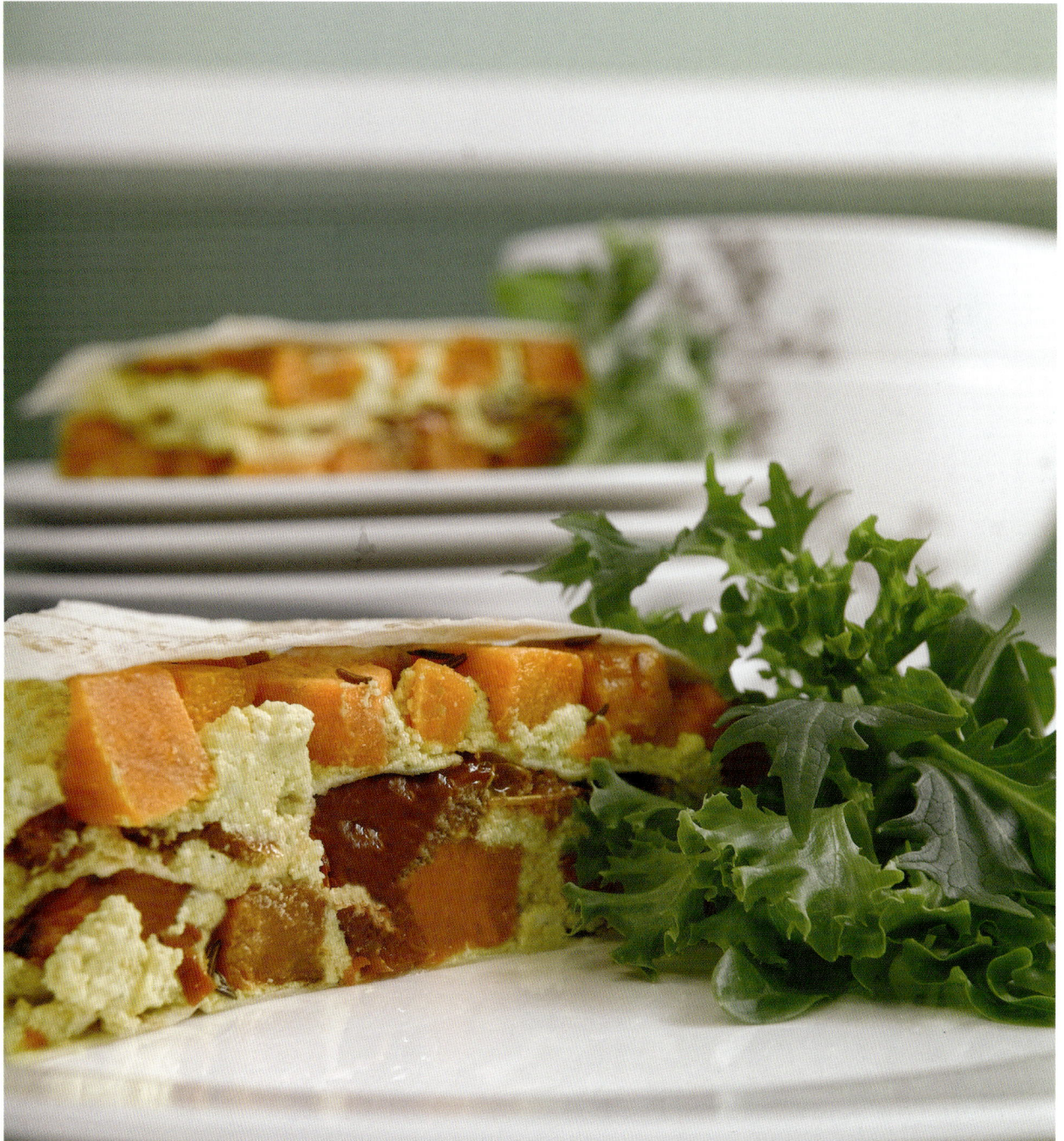

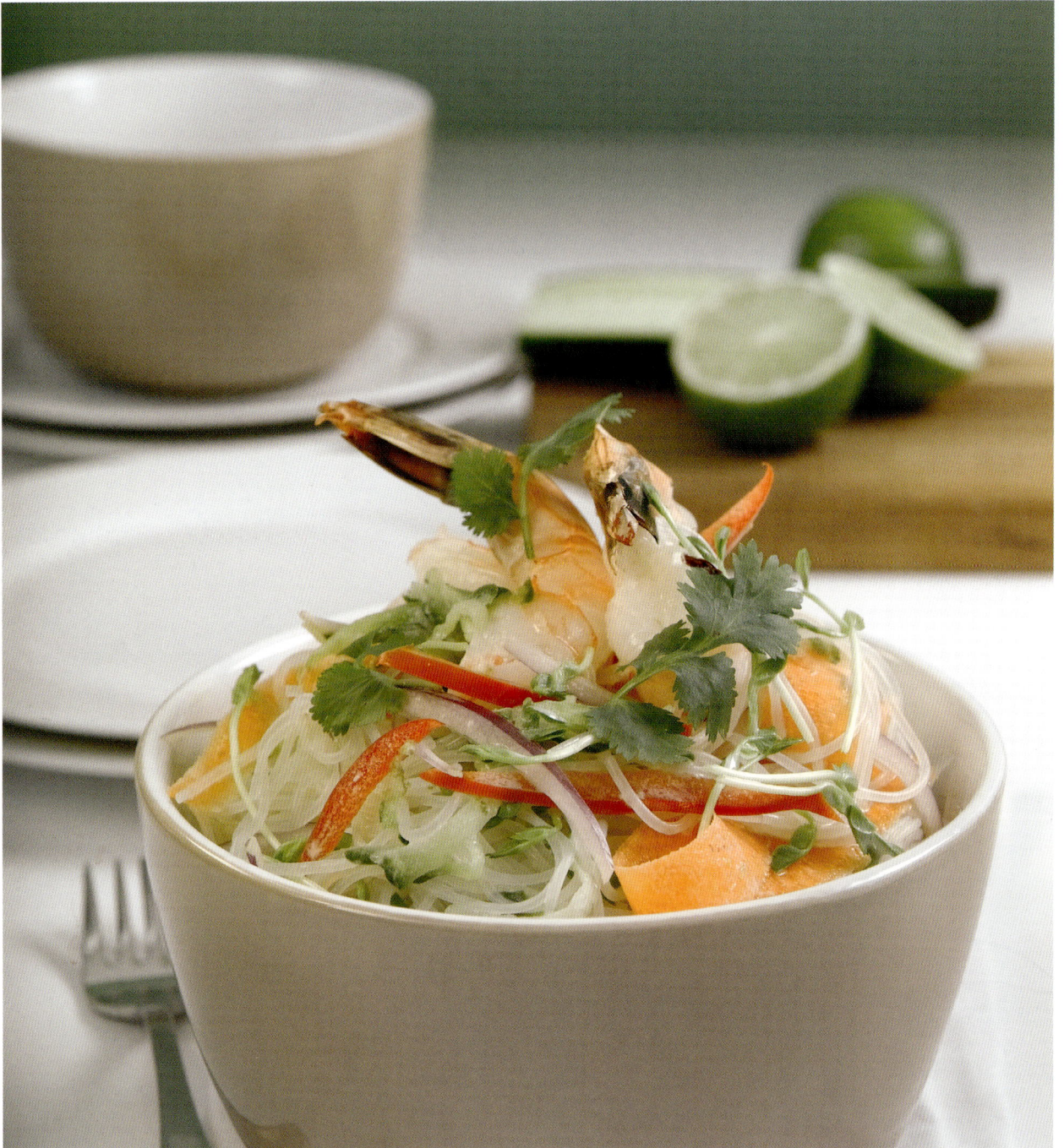

Prawn Glass Noodle Salad

Preparation time: 20 minutes
Cooking time: 7 minutes
Serves: 4

300g medium cooked king prawns, peeled and deveined
125g dried bean thread noodles
75g carrot, peeled and cut into strips
75g Lebanese cucumber, shredded, seeds removed
1 small red onion, finely sliced
60g snow pea sprouts
60g red capsicum, finely sliced
coriander leaves to garnish

For the dressing

1 tablespoon natural pineapple juice
1 tablespoon lime zest, finely grated
3 tablespoons lime juice
1 tablespoon raw sugar
60 ml (¼ cup) lite coconut milk
1 tablespoon fish sauce (nam pla)

Nutritional information: amounts per serve	
Energy (kJ)	1290
Protein (g)	23
Total Fat (g)	10.3
Saturated Fat (g)	6.5
Total Carbohydrate (g)	28
Sugars (g)	9.5
Fibre (g)	4.5
Sodium (mg)	1070
G.I.	low

1. Chop the prawns into halves or smaller pieces if you like.
2. Put the noodles into a large bowl and pour boiling water over to cover them. Let sit for 5–7 minutes then strain and run under cold water to stop cooking. Tip the noodles into a mixing bowl and allow to cool. Add all the other ingredients, except for the coriander leaves, and toss gently using your hands.
3. Make the dressing by combining all the ingredients. Stir well to ensure the sugar is dissolved. Pour the dressing over the noodle ingredients and toss gently. Top with the coriander leaves and serve.

These noodles are sometimes called mung bean noodles. You can replace them with rice vermicelli noodles if you like.

Red Capsicum and Mixed Vegetable Stew

Preparation time: 10 minutes
Cooking time: 30 minutes
Serves: 4

1 cup low-sodium, no-added-sugar tomatoes, crushed
1 cup low-sodium vegetable stock or water
200g red capsicum, chopped
150g red onion, chopped
125g peeled carrot, chopped
125g celery, chopped
125g mushrooms, chopped
10g garlic, chopped
1 large red chilli, chopped with seeds in
1 tablespoon parsley, chopped
1 teaspoon coriander powder
1 teaspoon ground black pepper

1. Bring the tomatoes and stock to the boil. Add the other ingredients except for the parsley, coriander and pepper. Simmer for 25 minutes, stirring regularly.
2. Check to see whether the vegetables are cooked after 25 minutes. Add the parsley, coriander and pepper. Cook for another 5–7 minutes and serve.

I use this stew in so many ways. It makes a great lunch and is delicious served as a gravy with barbecued lamb or beef. I have used it under grilled fish and on its own, with some wholemeal pasta. This versatile dish can be frozen in portions to suit your needs.

Nutritional information: amounts per serve	
Energy (kJ)	280
Protein (g)	4
Total Fat (g)	0.5
Saturated Fat (g)	0.1
Total Carbohydrate (g)	9
Sugars (g)	8
Fibre (g)	5
Sodium (mg)	60
G.I.	n/a

Minted Prawns with Rocket and Pink Grapefruit Salsa

Preparation time: 25 minutes
Serves: 4

2 medium pink grapefruit
24 medium cooked king prawns, peeled and deveined
2 tablespoons grapefruit juice (from the peeling process)
1 cup crisp mint leaves
1 small sweet green chilli, finely chopped
8 blanched asparagus spears, tips only
1 teaspoon green Tabasco
1 teaspoon raw sugar
2 tablespoons hazelnut oil
100g crisp rocket leaves, washed and ripped into pieces
¼ cup roasted salted cashews, chopped

1. Peel the grapefruits and break into segments over a bowl to catch the juice.
2. Chop the prawns into three pieces. Mix with grapefruit juice and mint leaves. Tumble and let sit for 20 minutes.
3. Mix the grapefruit segments, chili, asparagus, Tabasco, sugar and oil together. Let sit for 10 minutes.
4. Spread the rocket leaves onto four dinner plates and spoon on the salsa. Top with equal amounts of prawn pieces, sprinkle on cashews and spoon over any juices that may be left.

This salad is so good for lunch or as a starter for dinner. Serve with good, low GI bread and it will keep you filled up longer.

Nutritional information: amounts per serve	
Energy (kJ)	820
Protein (g)	4.5
Total Fat (g)	15
Saturated Fat (g)	2
Total Carbohydrate (g)	11
Sugars (g)	8
Fibre (g)	2.5
Sodium (mg)	80
G.I.	low

Smoked Trout, Hummus and Avocado Roti

Preparation time: 5–10 minutes
Cooking time: 5 minutes
Serves: 4

4 traditional Indian roti breads
1 cup hummus (store purchased or made with recipe on page 15 in Basics)
2 cups flaked, smoked trout flesh, bones and skin removed
1 large avocado, deseeded, skinned and cut into slices
60g rocket
2 tablespoons tarragon vinegar
1 tablespoon ground black pepper

1. Lightly brown the roti breads under the griller on both sides. When done, put onto four individual plates and spread equal quantities of hummus over each one.
2. Spread the trout evenly over the hummus and top with avocado slices.
3. Toss the rocket in the vinegar and arrange over the avocado; sprinkle on the pepper evenly and serve.

I have come to adore the flavour of smoked trout—actually anything that is smoked. I grew up on smoked haddock as we lived in a small country town and fresh, saltwater fish was a luxury rarely seen. Mum mastered cooking the smoked haddock then and endeared me to the flavour of smoked fish.

Nutritional information: amounts per serve	
Energy (kJ)	1980
Protein (g)	30
Total Fat (g)	25
Saturated Fat (g)	5
Total Carbohydrate (g)	26
Sugars (g)	2
Fibre (g)	10
Sodium (mg)	380
G.I.	medium

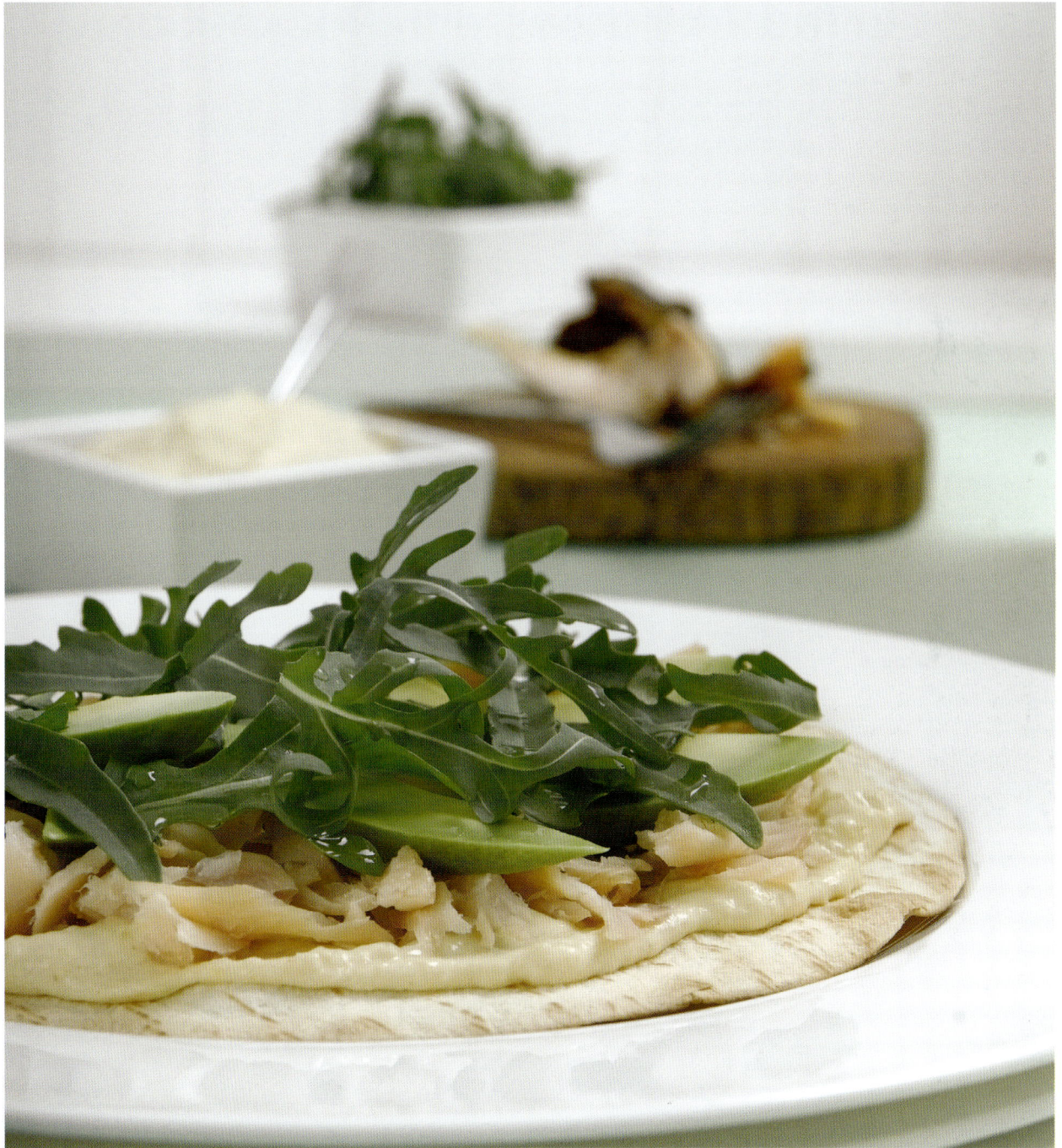

Tuna-Stuffed Tomatoes with Rocket Salad

Preparation time: 20 minutes
Serves: 4

4 ripe firm tomatoes, around 100g each
4 tablespoons canned/bottled corn kernels
3 tablespoons red onion, diced
185g drained tuna in spring water
2 tablespoons parsley, chopped
1 tablespoon coarsely ground black pepper
2 tablespoons lemon juice
8 cooked and skinned baby beetroots , quartered

For the salad

2 tablespoons linseed oil
1 teaspoon seeded mustard
3 tablespoons lemon juice
1 tablespoon tomato flesh, diced
50g rocket leaves
30g mixed leaves

1. Cut the tops from the tomatoes and keep. Ease the flesh out of the tomatoes with a sharp teaspoon and roughly chop. Cut the flesh from the tops, roughly chop and add.
2. Mix the corn, onion, tuna, parsley, pepper, lemon juice and tomato flesh. Spoon the mixture into each tomato and press it in with the back of the spoon. Cover with cling wrap and store in refrigerator until ready to serve.
3. Whisk the oil and mustard, add lemon juice and 1 tablespoon tomato flesh.
4. Add the rocket and mixed leaves to the dressing and toss to coat. Put an equal amount into the centre of four plates and add beetroot pieces around the edge of the salad leaves. Sit a tomato in the middle of the leaves, put the top on each one and serve.

Any leftover filling makes an excellent sandwich the next day. The tuna mixture develops such beautiful flavour that I make the mixture the day before stuffing the tomatoes.

Nutritional information: amounts per serve	
Energy (kJ)	880
Protein (g)	15
Total Fat (g)	11
Saturated Fat (g)	1.1
Total Carbohydrate (g)	11
Sugars (g)	9
Fibre (g)	4
Sodium (mg)	120
G.I.	low

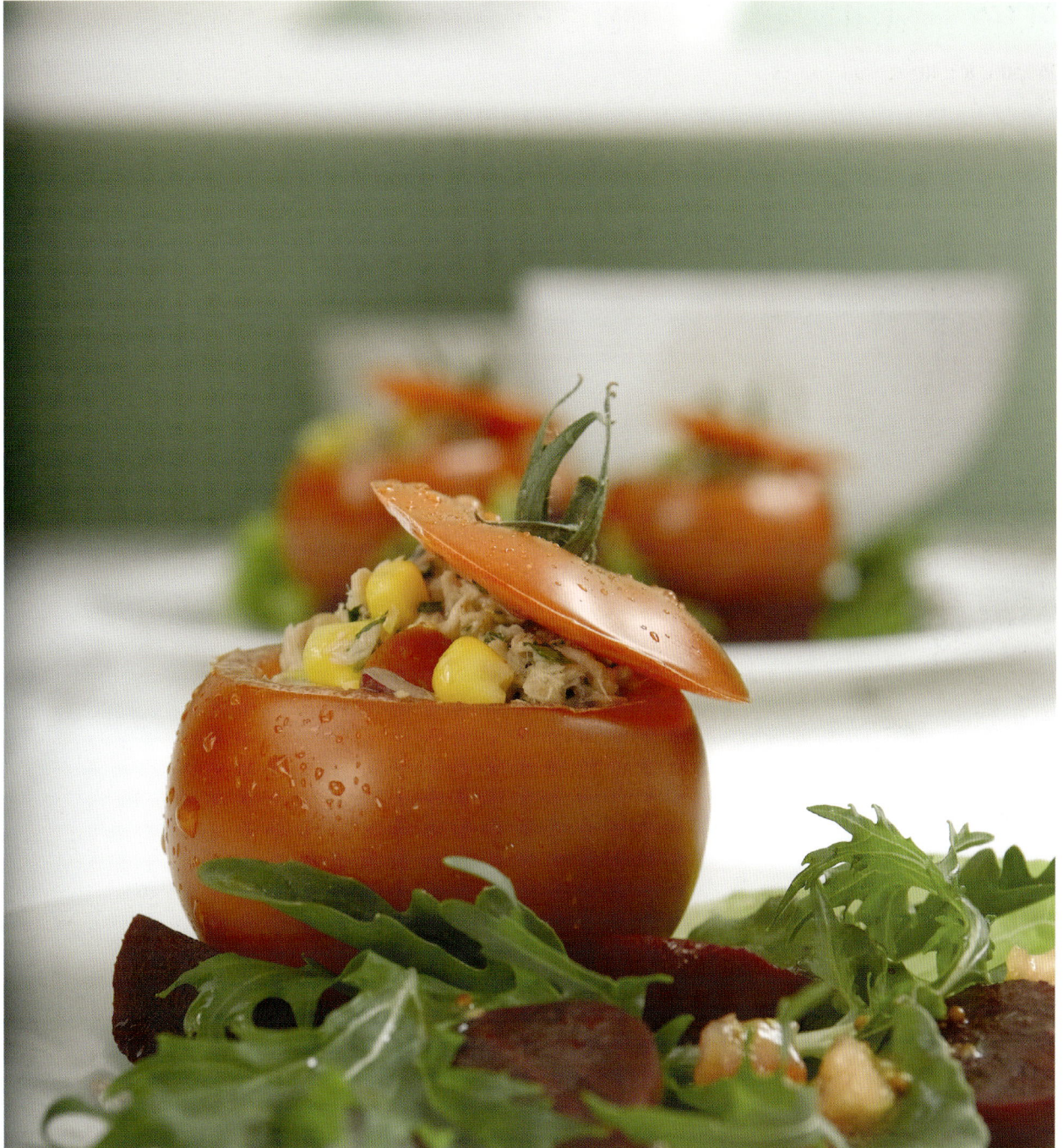

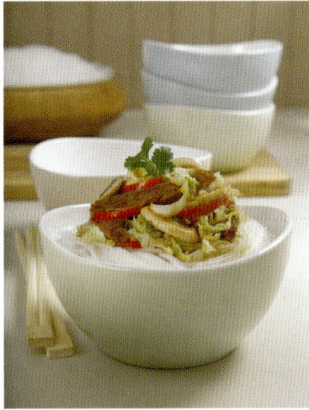 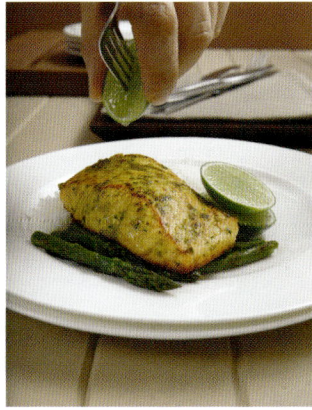 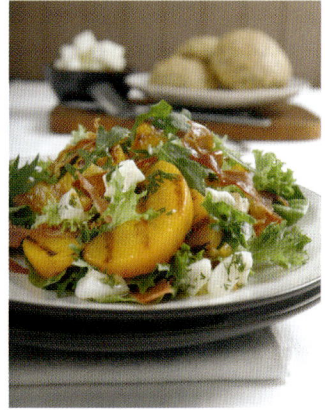

DINNER

As much as I try to make lunch my main intake of food, I generally end up with dinner as my main meal. There are lots of reasons and I think you would know them all—the busy day, the lack of time to cook during the day—and, of course, the evening being a time to catch up with family and friends and to relax.

I have tried to make the dinner recipes fit that bill. I have also added a couple of fancy dishes that may do for the next DP (dinner party). By the way, some of the lunch recipes can be used for dinner too, so don't forget to look at them if you want more inspiration. I do eat smaller portions for dinner these days and love fish or vegetarian for the evening meal.

If I have a more complicated dinner, I always finish with a piece of fruit. If I have a lighter dish—say a salad or similar—I treat myself to a dessert from the dessert section: a scoop of low-fat ice cream or a piece of my wonderful boiled fruit cake (which I have on hand all the time because it is so easy to make).

Dinner is an important meal and most of us have to have a big meal after working through the day. Do watch how much you have to eat and eat early if you can, to let the food digest. A good walk after dinner is best. After that you'll feel relaxed and ready to rest.

Barbecued Steak with Kumara Colcannon

Preparation time: 25 minutes
Cooking time: 5–10 minutes
Serves: 4

Preheat barbecue
4 x 200g lean sirloin steak
2 tablespoons green pepper corns
spray canola oil
4 cups green cabbage, roughly chopped
¼ cup skim milk
2 cups kumara sweet potato, steamed and roughly mashed
½ cup onion, roughly chopped
¼ teaspoon ground white pepper
200g green beans, topped

1. Preheat barbecue. Trim the beef of all fat and press the peppercorns into both sides of each steak. Refrigerate until nearly ready to use. Steak must be brought to room temperature before barbecuing, so take from the refrigerator at least 20 minutes for use.
2. Spray a pan with a little oil and cook the cabbage over medium heat until lightly browned.
3 Tip the milk into a saucepan and add the kumara and onion. Stir over medium to hot heat and stir in the cooked cabbage. Add the white pepper and combine. Keep warm.
4. Cook the steaks to your liking. I cook these on the flat plate and do not spray with oil. Make sure the steaks are cooked and rested for at least 5 minutes before serving. This way the juices are set and do not bleed onto the other food on the plate.
5. Plunge the beans into boiling water and bring back to the boil to cook to your liking. Drain and pile into the centre of a heated dinner plate. Spoon the kumara colcannon (mash) evenly over the beans so that some of the beans are showing. Top with cooked steak and serve.

Nutritional information: amounts per serve	
Energy (kJ)	850
Protein (g)	15
Total Fat (g)	4
Saturated Fat(g)	1.5
Total Carbohydrate (g)	23
Sugar (g)	9
Fibre (g)	7
Sodium (mg)	64
G.I.	low

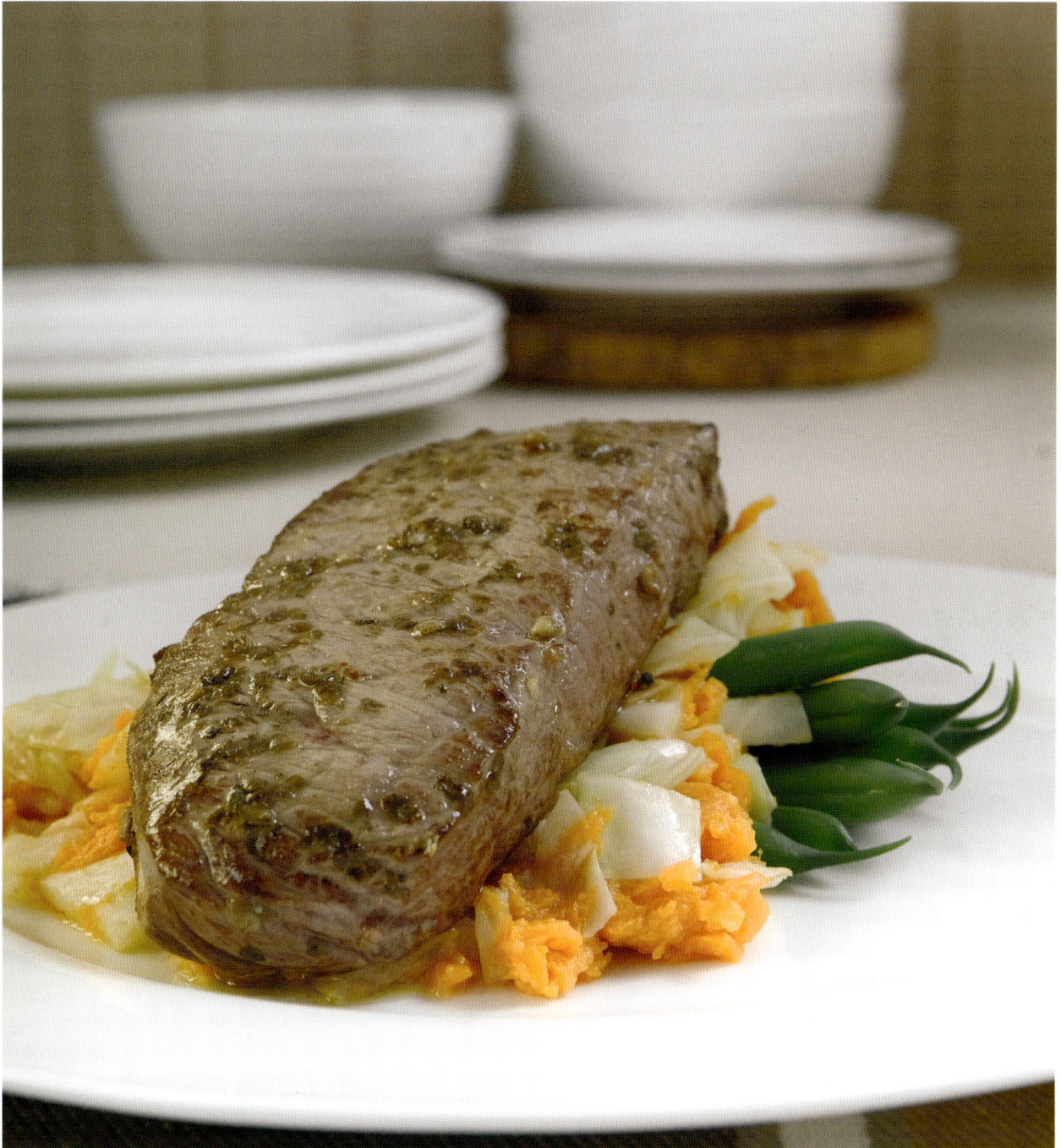

Buckwheat Pancakes and Caponata

Preparation time: 15 minutes
Cooking time: 60 minutes
Serves: 4

For the pancakes see recipe in Basics (page 22)

For the caponata
1 cup low sodium vegetable stock
1 large onion, peeled and diced roughly
2 medium eggplants, diced into 3cm pieces
1 cup diced celery

½ cup green olives, seeded and chopped
2 cups tomatoes, diced
¼ cup drained capers
½ cup lemon juice and zest of that lemon
1 tablespoon honey (yellow box if possible)
2 bay leaves
Basil leaves for garnish

1. Prepare the pancake batter first. Leave to sit for one hour before use.
2. Preheat oven to 180°C (fan-forced 160°C). Put all the caponata ingredients into a casserole dish and cook in the oven for 1 hour. Stir occasionally, when done cool and refrigerate if not using immediately. The mixture needs to be dryish for this recipe. If you have too much juice, either spoon some out or simmer on top of the stove to reduce liquid.
3. Make and cook the pancakes as per recipe and keep warm.
4. To serve, lay out the pancakes and spoon the caponata down the centre. Roll the pancakes around the caponata filling and place on plates. This is best done with warm caponata, reheated in the microwave. Decorate with ripped basil leaves.

These are just great at room temperature too. If you want to slightly heat them, put them into a hot oven for 5 minutes and they are ready to eat.

The caponata freezes well, if you have any left over, or can be refrigerated for 7 days.

Nutritional information: amounts per serve	
Energy (kJ)	1230
Protein (g)	13
Total Fat (g)	4.5
Saturated Fat (g)	1.2
Total Carbohydrate (g)	45
Sugars (g)	22
Fibre (g)	9
Sodium (mg)	540
G.I.	low

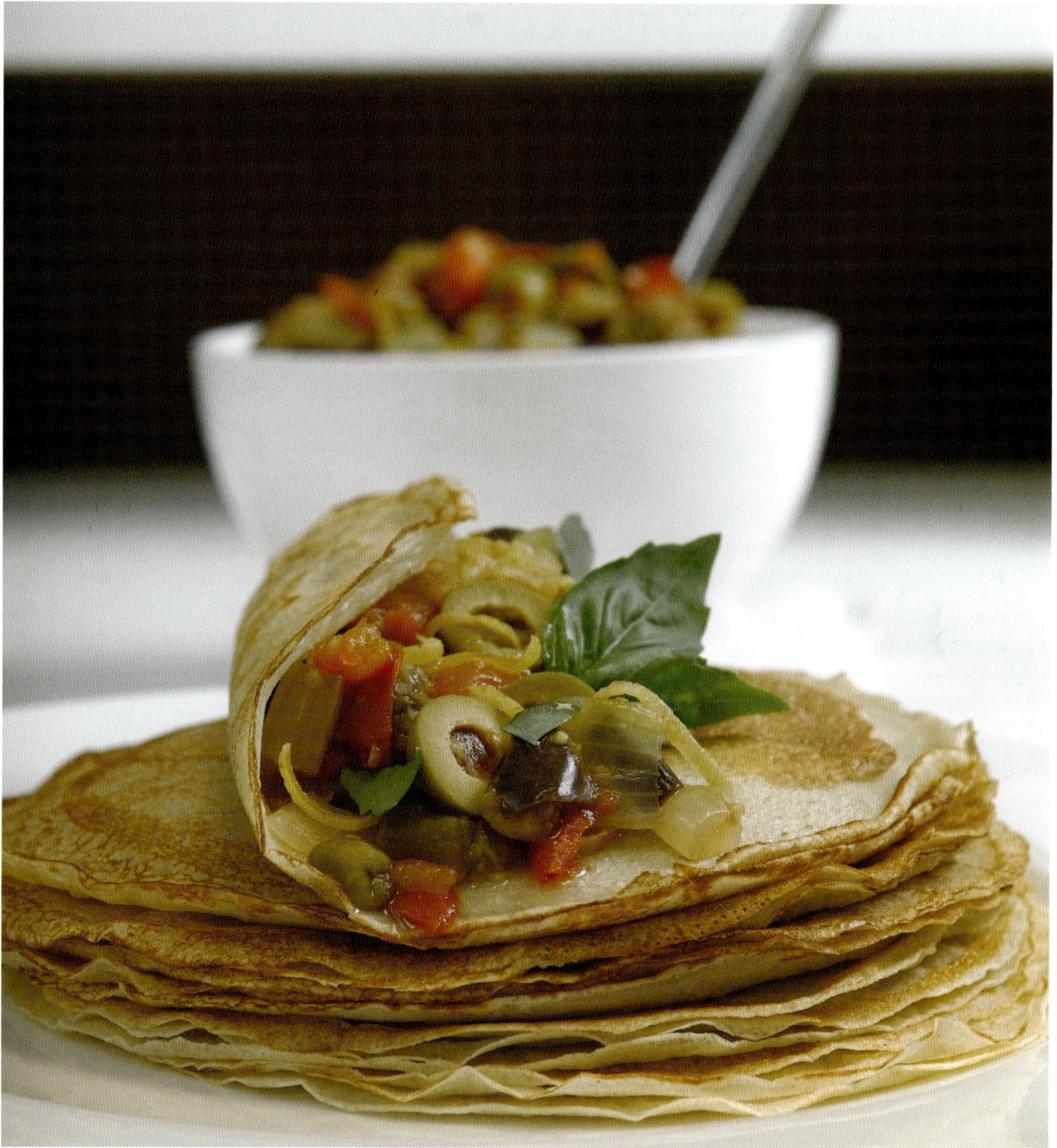

Chermoula Atlantic Salmon and Charred Asparagus

Preparation time: 10 minutes
Cooking time: 5 minutes
Serves: 4

4 x 150g Atlantic salmon steaks, skin removed
½ cup chermoula (see Basics page 14)
spray canola oil
24 asparagus spears, trimmed
4 lime cheeks

1. Put the salmon steaks into a flattish tray, skin side down and tip over the chermoula. Pat it onto the fish and let sit for 10 minutes in the refrigerator.
2. To cook, preheat the barbecue flat plate to medium. Lift the fish from the tray and shake it carefully to avoid removing all the rub. Lightly spray the flesh side with oil and put onto the grill plate.
3. Lightly spray the asparagus and lay it on the plate too. If you have an open-slat char-grill, use that to cook the asparagus, but do watch it and turn regularly as it burns easily.
4. Salmon is best cooked to medium. Turn the salmon after 2 minutes having sprayed the other side. The fish will finish cooking very quickly.
5. Evenly divide the asparagus onto individual plates, top with the fish and decorate with a lime cheek. Serve with a cooked carbohydrate of your choice. I suggest steamed potatoes or basmati rice.

Atlantic salmon is so good to eat and so nutritious. The flavour is big and the omega-3 factor makes it even more attractive.
   When trimming the asparagus, you remove the woody white bit at the bottom. This breaks off easily where the white meets the green.

Nutritional information: amounts per serve	
Energy (kJ)	1030
Protein (g)	31
Total Fat (g)	11
Saturated Fat (g)	2.5
Total Carbohydrate (g)	2
Sugars (g)	2
Fibre (g)	4
Sodium (mg)	330
G.I.	n/a

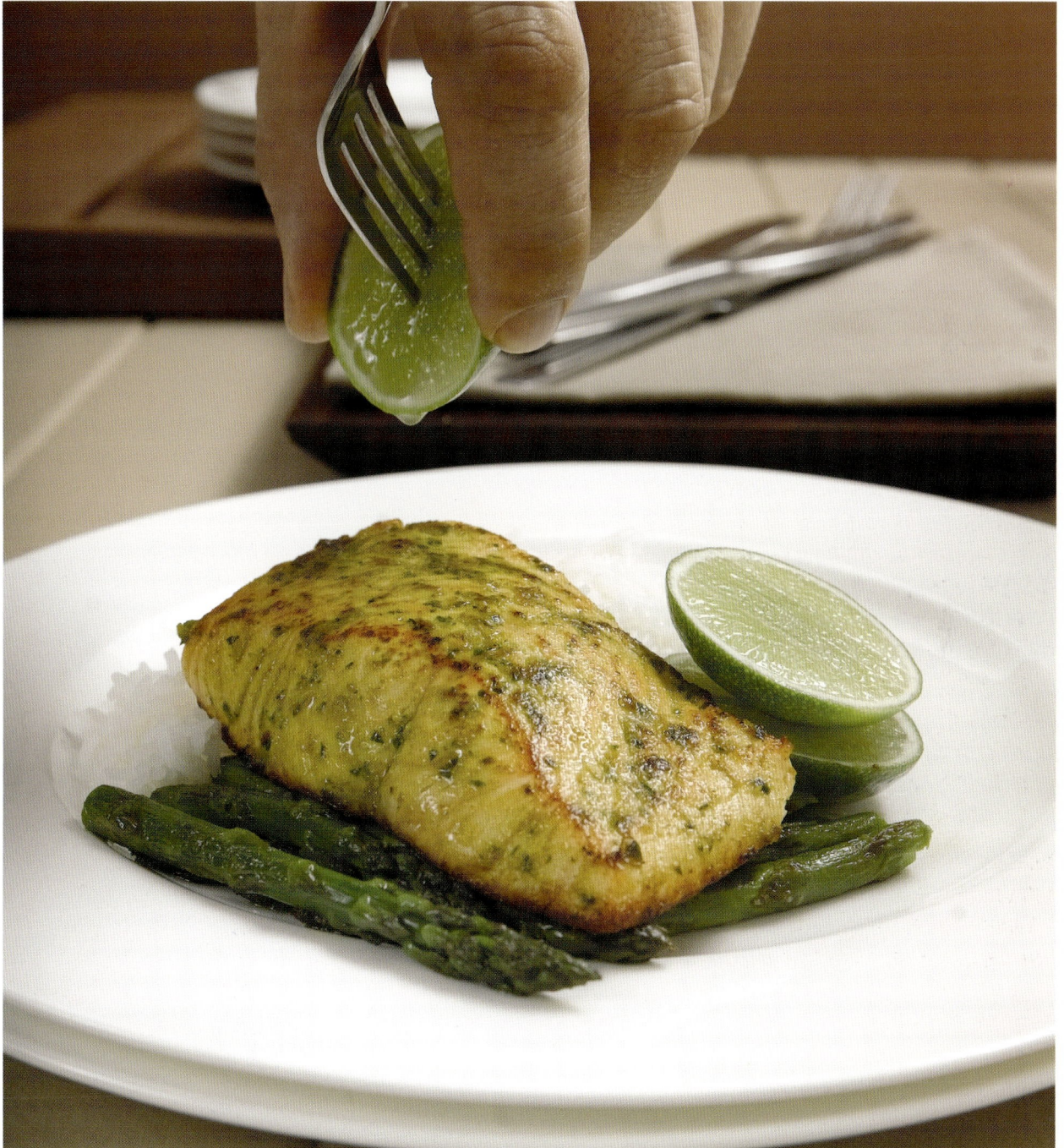

Chicken Choi Bao

Preparation time: 10 minutes
Cooking time: 15 minutes
Serves: 4

500g chicken, minced
1 tablespoon vegetable oil
1 small brown onion, finely chopped
4 cloves garlic, peeled and finely chopped
¼ cup hoi sin sauce
100g water chestnuts, drained and roughly chopped
1 small bunch fresh coriander, leaves only and finely broken
8 medium size lettuce cups, washed and crisped
Cooked brown or basmati rice

For the sauce
2 tablespoons rice vinegar
3 tablespoons Tamari light soy sauce
1 small red chilli, seeds in and minced

Nutritional information: amounts per serve	
Energy (kJ)	1380
Protein (g)	26
Total Fat (g)	17
Saturated Fat (g)	4
Total Carbohydrate (g)	16
Sugars (g)	13
Fibre (g)	5
Sodium (mg)	920
G.I.	medium

1. Check the chicken to ensure all fat is removed.
2. Bring the oil to smoking point over high heat and add the onion and garlic. Stir and add the chicken mince. Use the back of a large spoon or a wok spatula to mash the meat so it does not go lumpy. Pour in the hoi sin and add the water chestnuts. Cook for 10 minutes stirring occasionally.
3. Make the sauce by combining all ingredients.
4. Stir the coriander into the chicken and serve in a large bowl in the middle of the table with the lettuce cups and sauce to one side. Boiled, long grain rice always sets off this dish. I generally use brown rice but basmati is fine.

You can substitute the rice vinegar with regular white vinegar.

Chicken, Wilted Spinach and Curried Chickpeas

Preparation time: 15 minutes
Cooking time: 45 minutes
Serves: 4

4 x 125g skinless chicken breasts, cut into medallions
2 spring onions, chopped
1 tablespoon linseed oil
½ medium onion, finely chopped
½ medium carrot, finely chopped
2 tablespoons Indian curry powder
400g canned pre cooked chickpeas, drained
2 cups water
200g baby spinach leaves

Nutritional information: amounts per serve	
Energy (kJ)	1490
Protein (g)	36
Total Fat (g)	14
Saturated Fat (g)	3
Total Carbohydrate (g)	17
Sugars (g)	3
Fibre (g)	9
Sodium (mg)	350
G.I.	low

1. Ensure all fat is removed from the chicken medallions. Heat enough water to poach the chicken, add chicken and spring onion and simmer for 10 minutes. Turn off the heat until ready to use.
2. Heat linseed oil and lightly fry the onion and carrot pieces. Tip in the curry powder and stir. Add the drained chickpeas and stir to coat with the curry mixture. Pour in the 2 cups water, bring to the boil then reduce to a simmer and cook for 30 minutes. You may need more water, depending on the saucepan you use.
3. Reheat the poaching stock, simmer the chicken slices to cook through: around 3–5 minutes. Do this in batches, depending on your pan size. Keep slices warm if this is the case.
4. In another saucepan bring ½ cup chicken poaching liquid to the boil. Tip in the spinach and stir to allow it to wilt/break down. Do not overcook or you will lose the colour and nutritional value. Drain well and keep warm.
5. Serve by putting equal amounts of chickpeas into the centre of four deep-welled plates. Top with spinach, then equal amounts of chicken slices. Spoon over some of the chicken poaching liquid and serve immediately. Serve with good bread.

If you are not in a bread mood when you have this yummy dish, you can always have a good carbohydrate dessert instead.

This delicious chickpea recipe is best made the day before, to let the flavour meld.

I often buy larger chicken breasts for this recipe and cut them into medallions for easier cooking.

Chilli Lamb Skewers and Asian Slaw

Preparation time: 15 minutes
Cooking time: 5 minutes
Serves: 4

500g lean lamb strips
4 stainless skewers or bamboo skewers that have been soaked in water for 15 minutes
½ teaspoon chilli powder
4 cups Chinese cabbage, shredded
½ cup finely sliced spring onions (aka shallots)
½ cup red capsicum, diced
50g snow pea sprouts
¼ cup Tamari low salt soy sauce
1 tablespoon green ginger, minced
1 small red chilli, seeds in and minced
1 teaspoon sesame oil
1 teaspoon raw sugar
2 tablespoon lime juice
4 lime cheeks

Nutritional information: amounts per serve	
Energy (kJ)	910
Protein (g)	30
Total Fat (g)	6
Saturated Fat (g)	2
Total Carbohydrate (g)	7
Sugars (g)	6
Fibre (g)	3
Sodium (mg)	670
G.I.	n/a

1. Buy the lamb already in strips if you like. I cut mine down from the mini roast so that I can control the amount of fat and trim accordingly. I cut them into strips about 2cm (¾in) thick and 2cm (¾in) wide. Thread equal amounts onto skewers in an 'S' shape. Sprinkle evenly with the chilli and let sit for 5 minutes.
2. Make the slaw by combining the cabbage, onion, capsicum and snow pea sprouts. In a separate container, mix the soy, ginger, chilli, oil, sugar and lime juice. Stir well, pour over the cabbage mix and toss well. Serve as soon as possible.
3. Grill, pan fry or barbecue the lamb, which will cook in 5 minutes, or leave longer for well done.
4. Serve each skewer of lamb on top of equal amounts of slaw and with a lime cheek on each plate.

Curried Chicken and Steamed Pearl Barley

Preparation time: 10 minutes
Cooking time: 40 minutes
Serves: 4

500g chicken thigh meat
½ cup low-sodium chicken stock
1 onion (100g), roughly chopped
1 cup (120g) celery, chopped
3 tablespoons curry powder
(Sri Lankan Curry powder, page 21, or your favourite curry powder)
400g can no-added-salt tomatoes, crushed
500 ml (2 cups) low-sodium chicken stock
100g red lentils, washed
200g pearl barley, washed
2 cloves garlic, crushed
½ teaspoon white pepper

Nutritional information: amounts for whole recipe	
Energy (kJ)	2000
Protein (g)	38.5
Total Fat (g)	12
Saturated Fat (g)	3
Total Carbohydrate (g)	48
Sugars (g)	7
Fibre (g)	13
Sodium (mg)	760
G.I.	low

1. Cut the chicken into even pieces, ensuring all fat has been removed.
2. Heat the stock and add the onion and celery. Stir over high heat for 2 minutes, stir in curry powder and cook for another minute.
3. Add the chicken to lightly colour, then tip in the tomatoes and chicken stock. Simmer for 30 minutes then stir in the lentils and cook for another 5–8 minutes.
4. Cook the barley while the curry simmers by putting it into a large saucepan and covering with water (see note below). Bring to the boil then reduce to very low heat. Cook with the lid on until the barley is done and soft. Stir in the garlic and pepper.
5. Serve the curry, when done, over the barley and with minted no-fat yoghurt if you desire.

The barley is different and delicious. I could eat it on its own as a snack. Whole barley is the best, but takes longer to cook as it has more layers of husk left on each grain. The pearl barley takes 20 minutes, plus 5 minutes just sitting with the lid off. Use the rice absorption cooking method, which is one knuckle of water above the top of the rice … use your middle finger. I saw this at Brisbane Masterclass 2005 when Chef Peter Kuravita showed this method. He explained that all middle finger first knuckles are almost exactly the same size. Odd but true. Try it with whoever is around and you'll be as surprised as I was. This amount of uncooked barley makes 4 half cups of cooked barley.

No-Added-Fat Beef and Mushroom Stir-Fry

Preparation time: 20 minutes + time to marinate
Cooking time: 5–7 minutes
Serves: 4

600g lean steak
1 tablespoon red chilli (bottled or fresh), minced
1 tablespoon garlic, minced
¼ cup salt-reduced tamari soy sauce
1 cup sodium-reduced, no-fat beef stock
1 medium onion, cut into thin wedges
1 red capsicum, cut into strips
100g sliced mushroom, medium size
20g green ginger, grated
2 cups Chinese cabbage, sliced
200g cooked rice vermicelli noodles
1 cup coriander, leaves only

Nutritional information: amounts per serve	
Energy (kJ)	1240
Protein (g)	38
Total Fat (g)	8
Saturated Fat (g)	3
Total Carbohydrate (g)	16
Sugars (g)	3
Fibre (g)	3
Sodium (mg)	930
G.I.	low

1. Trim the beef of all fat, cut into fine strips and put in bowl with chilli, garlic and soy sauce. Turn well and leave to marinate for 20 minutes.
2. To cook, pour half the beef stock into a wok and bring to the boil over high heat. Add the onion and capsicum and stir-fry for 2 minutes. Drain the beef and add. If you have a small wok, you will need to do this in two batches after you have removed the vegetables with a slotted spoon. You need to leave stock in the base to stop the meat from sticking to the wok.
3. When the beef is lightly browned return the onion and capsicum to the wok then add the rest of the stock, mushrooms and ginger. Stir-fry for two minutes then add the cabbage and cook to combine.
4. Serve in individual bowls with the stir-fry spooned over the rice noodles and topped with ripped coriander leaves.

I use the salt-reduced tamari sauce, but you can find organic ones too. This sauce does not have any wheat in it, so is excellent for coeliacs.

Beef stock is available as a liquid or in dried cubes. Look for those that are low in salt. I have found Massel stock cubes and liquid to be the best for my purposes.

I always cut my own beef strips so that I know how fatty the meat is. You need to have lean meat, cut in fine strips for quick cooking.

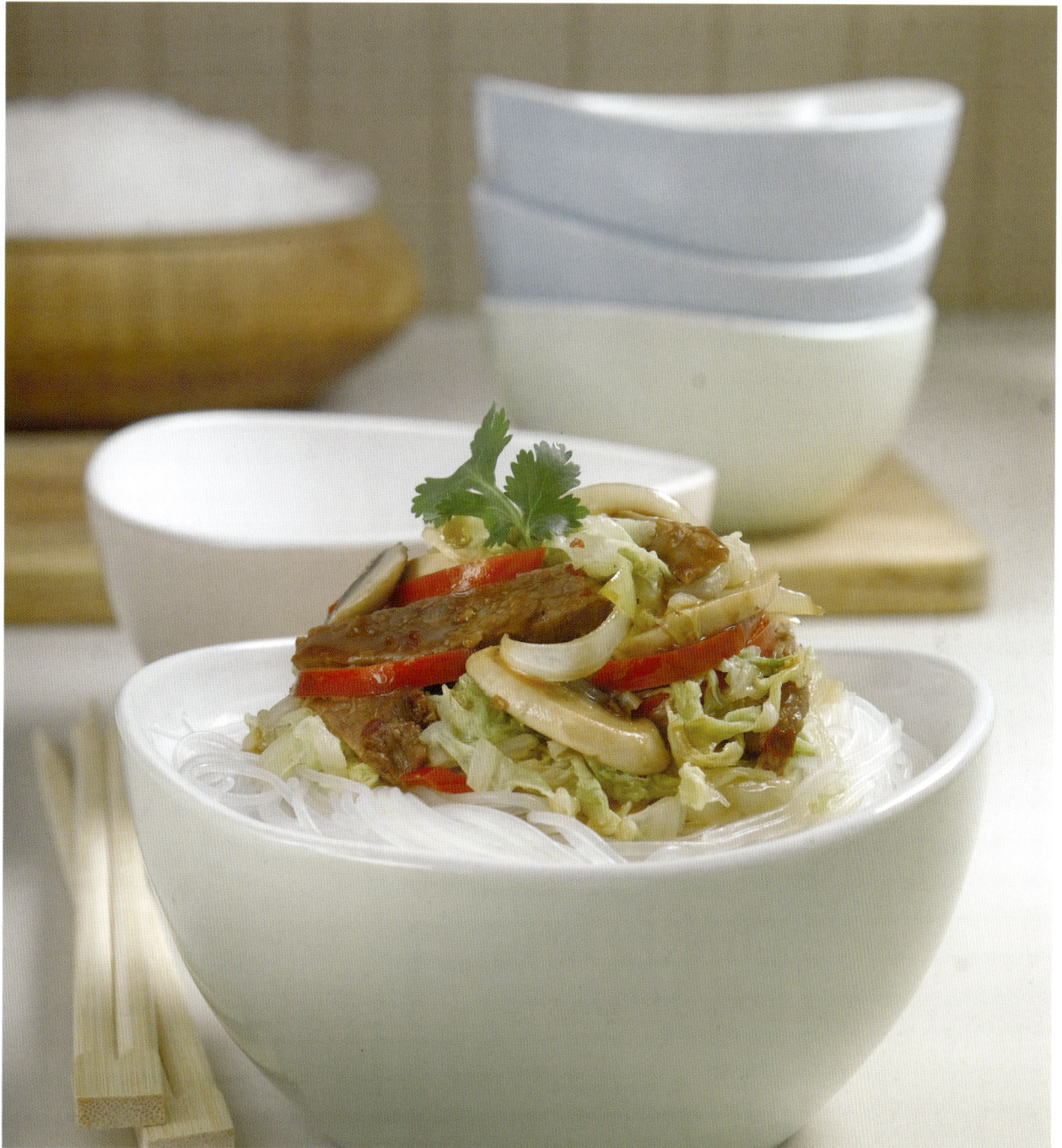

Olive Parsley Lamb with White Turnip Stew

Preparation time: 20 minutes
Cooking time: 45 minutes
Serves: 4

2 x 200g mini lamb roasts
1½ tablespoons smooth French mustard
4 tablespoons olive parsley paste (see Basics page 14)
120g onion, roughly chopped
150g celery, roughly diced
400g white turnip, roughly diced
vegetable stock, made from 1 vegetable stock cube, around 500 ml (2 cups)
½ teaspoon ground white pepper

1. Pre heat oven to 180°C (fan-forced 160°C) Trim all fat from the lamb. Mix the mustard with olive parsley paste and smear over the top lamb. Leave to sit for 5 minutes.
2. Put a cooling rack onto a baking tray and place the lamb onto the rack. Cook for 40 minutes or until done to your liking. Remove from oven to rest for 10 minutes before slicing.
3. Meanwhile cook the onion, celery and turnips in the vegetable stock. Just cover the mixed vegetables and simmer until done: 15–20 minutes. Add the white pepper towards the end of the cooking.
4. Serve vegetables onto dinner plates. Slice the lamb roasts around 2cm thick and serve equal amounts of it on top of the vegetables.

Watch the white pepper as it builds in intensity as it cooks and lingers on the palate.

I just love the white turnip stew and I use the leftovers on rye toast (or similar) for breakfast next morning (if there is any left that is).

Nutritional information: amounts per serve	
Energy (kJ)	710
Protein (g)	23
Total Fat (g)	4
Saturated Fat (g)	1.7
Total Carbohydrate (g)	7
Sugars (g)	6
Fibre (g)	4.5
Sodium (mg)	400
G.I.	n/a

Tuna and Hummus Brochette with Pink Grapefruit Salad

Preparation time: 20 minutes
Cooking time: 10 minutes
Serves: 4

4 x 150g tuna steaks
1 tablespoon mustard seed oil
½ tablespoon ground black pepper
1–2 grapefruit
100g mixed lettuce leaves
4 thick slices sour dough bread
spray canola oil
2 cloves garlic, peeled
250g beetroot pinto bean hummus (see Basics page 12)

Nutritional information: amounts per serve	
Energy (kJ)	1955
Protein (g)	46
Total Fat (g)	18
Saturated Fat (g)	5
Total Carbohydrate (g)	27
Sugars (g)	8
Fibre (g)	6
Sodium (mg)	380
G.I.	low

1. Put the tuna steaks into a glass bowl, tip in the oil and sprinkle in the pepper. Move the tuna around to coat with oil and pepper, then leave to sit for 10 minutes.
2. Make the salad by peeling the grapefruit first. Cut all the skin and pith away from the flesh and cut out each segment over a bowl to collect the juice. Put the leaves and segments into a bowl and add the collected juice. Toss gently.
3. Spray the bread lightly with oil and toast, grill or barbecue until browned and crisp. Rub the hot slices on one side with the garlic to infuse. Smear or spoon the beetroot hummus onto the garlic side of the bread and put onto individual serving plates.
4. Cook the tuna in a griddle pan or on a very hot barbeque until done to your liking (see note below). Top the beetroot brochette with the cooked tuna and place the tossed salad to one side. Spoon any juices over the top of the salad.

Tuna is a great source of omega-3 as well as being stunning to eat. I find it better not to cook tuna through as dries out. It is easy to watch while cooking as the side of each slice goes white as it cooks. You only need turn it over once, as the whitening approaches halfway up the side of the steak. As soon as the sides are completely white you are ready to serve medium to rare tuna.

Peach, Fetta and Prosciutto Salad with Lime and Lychee Dressing

Preparation time: 20 minutes
Cooking time: 10 minutes
Serves: 4

24 peach slices, canned and drained
spray canola oil
100g bag Mesculun lettuce leaves
200g fat-reduced fetta cheese, diced
1 tablespoon extra virgin olive oil
3 tablespoons fresh lime juice
60g canned lychees, cut into 1 cm cubes, drained
1 teaspoon dill, chopped
1 teaspoon green peppercorns
4 large slices prosciutto, grilled until crisp, cooled and crumbled

1. Lightly spray the peach slices with oil and barbecue on the open slat or cook in hot griddle pan until lightly browned. The slices mark very quickly so do 6 slices at a time. Leave to cool before adding to the leaves and cheese.
2. Make the dressing by whisking the oil slowly, whisk in the lime juice and stir in the lychee cubes, dill and peppercorns to taste.
3. Pour the dressing onto the peach and salad ingredients and toss gently. Sprinkle crumbled prosciutto over and serve.

Prosciutto can be quite salty, so you do not need salt in this recipe. To crisp the prosciutto, lay the slices on a cooling rack and place on a tray that will fit under the griller. Cook and let the fat drip onto the tray. Watch carefully as the slices cook quickly. Remove from heat, cool on kitchen towelling and crumble when cool.

Nutritional information: amounts per serve	
Energy (kJ)	1040
Protein (g)	16.5
Total Fat (g)	13.5
Saturated Fat (g)	5.7
Total Carbohydrate (g)	12
Sugars (g)	11
Fibre (g)	2.5
Sodium (mg)	970
G.I.	low

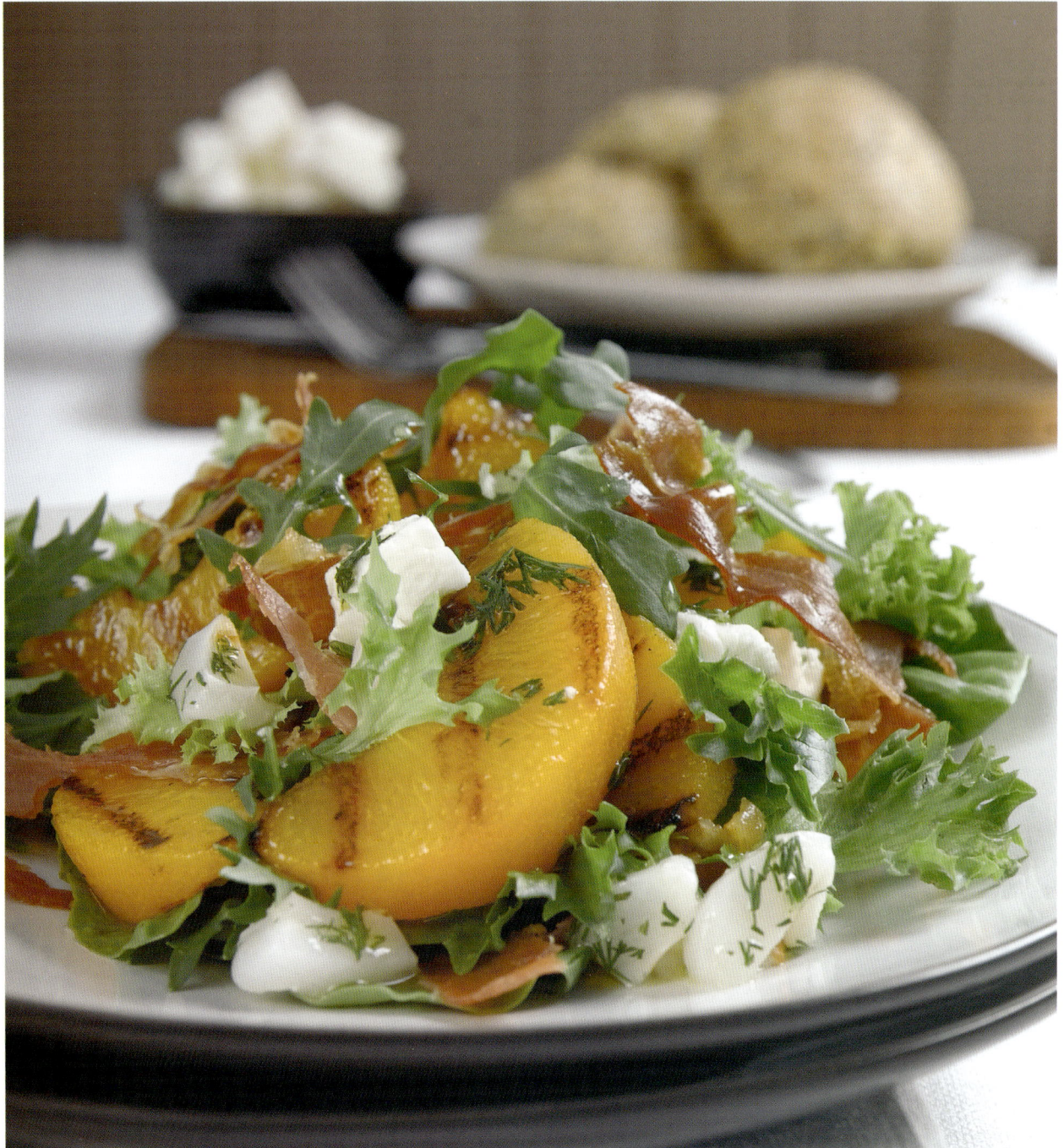

Spiced Yoghurt Pork Fillet and Pan-Fried Pears

Preparation time: 30 minutes
Cooking time: 20 minutes
Serves: 4

600g pork fillet, cut into medallions
150 ml (¾ cup) no-fat natural yoghurt
1 teaspoon smoked paprika powder
1 teaspoon fennel seeds, roughly crushed
1 teaspoon coriander powder
¼ medium onion, finely chopped
1 tablespoon minced fresh oregano
½ tablespoon mustard seed oil
lemon flavoured cracked peppercorns
8 canned pear halves, well drained
120g cooked silverbeet leaves

Nutritional information: amounts per serve	
Energy (kJ)	1200
Protein (g)	36.5
Total Fat (g)	6
Saturated Fat (g)	1.6
Total Carbohydrate (g)	19
Sugars (g)	18
Fibre (g)	3.5
Sodium (mg)	170
G.I.	low

1. Ensure all fat is removed from the pork medallions. Gently flatten them by pounding with the heel of your hand. Mix the yoghurt, paprika, fennel, coriander, onion and oregano well.
2. Preheat oven to 180°C (fan-forced160°C). Smear each piece of pork with the yogurt mixture and leave to sit for 15–30 minutes.
3. Place the pork into a baking tray and cook in the oven for 15 minutes until firm.
4. Heat the oil in a non-stick pan, sprinkle the pear halves with cracked pepper and pan-fry to golden brown.
5. Pile equal amounts of silverbeet onto the centre of each plate, top with equal quantities of pork and two pear halves each. Serve with a fat-free carbohydrate of your choice. I suggest steamed potatoes or basmati rice.

The thickness of each medallion will determine how long they take to cook. Mine were 4–5cm thick. I had eight of them and they cooked—well spaced on the tray—in the 15 minutes, which left them only just pink and the thinner ones not well done, but just right. It is okay to leave your pork fillet pink.

While testing another batch of this delicious pork dish, I found that the flavour improves if the pork is left in the yoghurt for 45 minutes, but this is dictated by the amount of time you have.

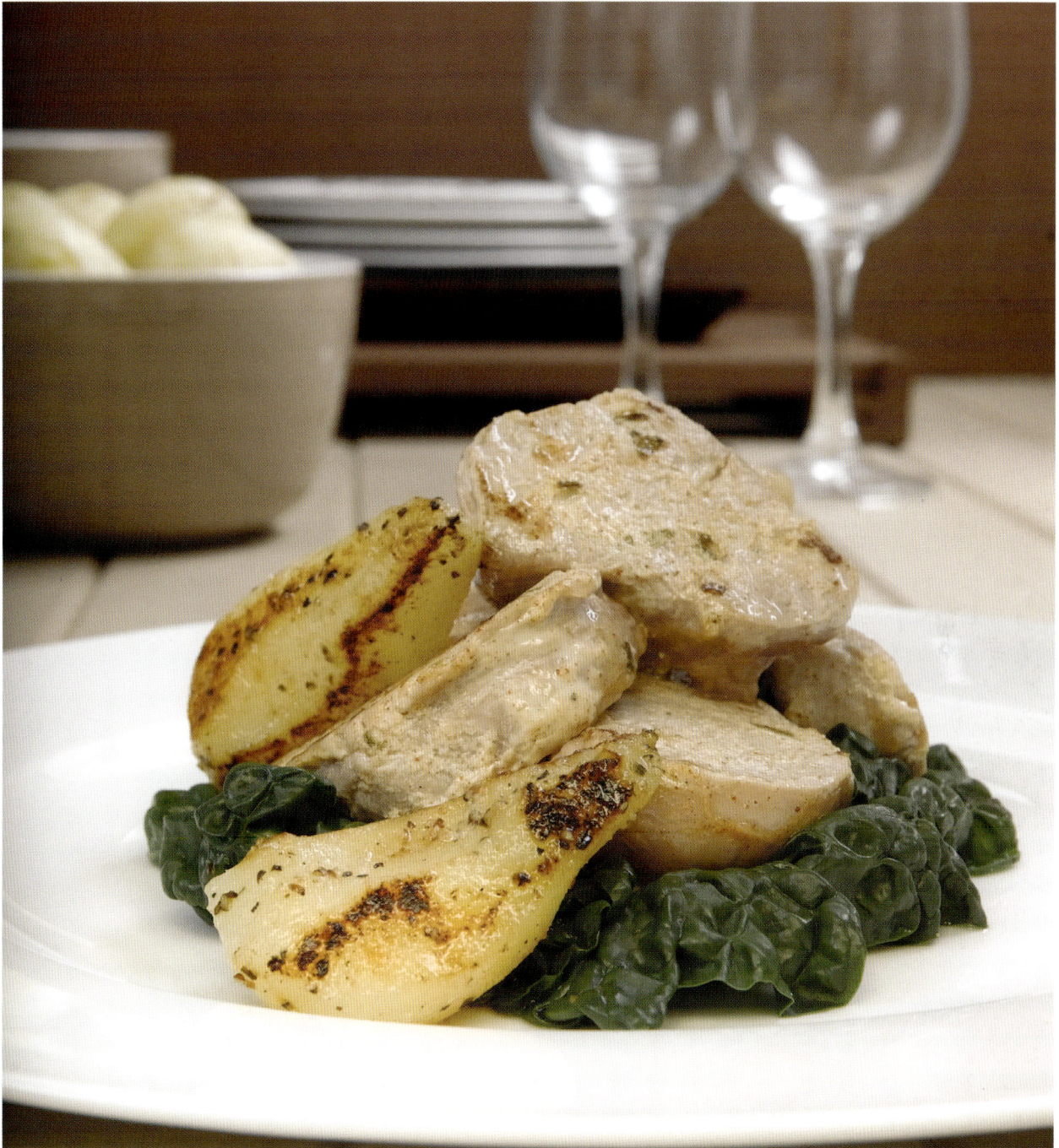

Tofu, Carrot and Lentil Strudel

Preparation time: 10 minutes
Cooking time: 45 minutes
Serves: 4

200g carrots, peeled and grated
150g firm tofu, diced
¾ cup precooked canned lentils, drained
10 pitted prunes
4 sheets filo pastry
spray canola oil
1 cup low-fat natural yoghurt
2 tablespoons fresh mint, chopped
1 teaspoon ground black pepper

1. Preheat oven 180ºC (fan-forced 160ºC). Combine the carrots, tofu and lentils and mix well.
2. Lay one sheet of pastry on the bench and spray lightly with oil. Top with another sheet and repeat until the pastry is all used.
3. Spoon the carrot filling down one side of the assembled pastry layers. Dot with prunes, roll and pull in the ends to make a sealed package. Lift onto a baking paper-lined baking tray, spray with a light coating of oil and bake until browned and crisp, about 30–40 minutes.

Nutritional information: amounts per serve	
Energy (kJ)	860
Protein (g)	12
Total Fat (g)	4
Saturated Fat (g)	0.5
Total Carbohydrate (g)	27
Sugars (g)	13
Fibre (g)	5
Sodium (mg)	290
G.I.	low

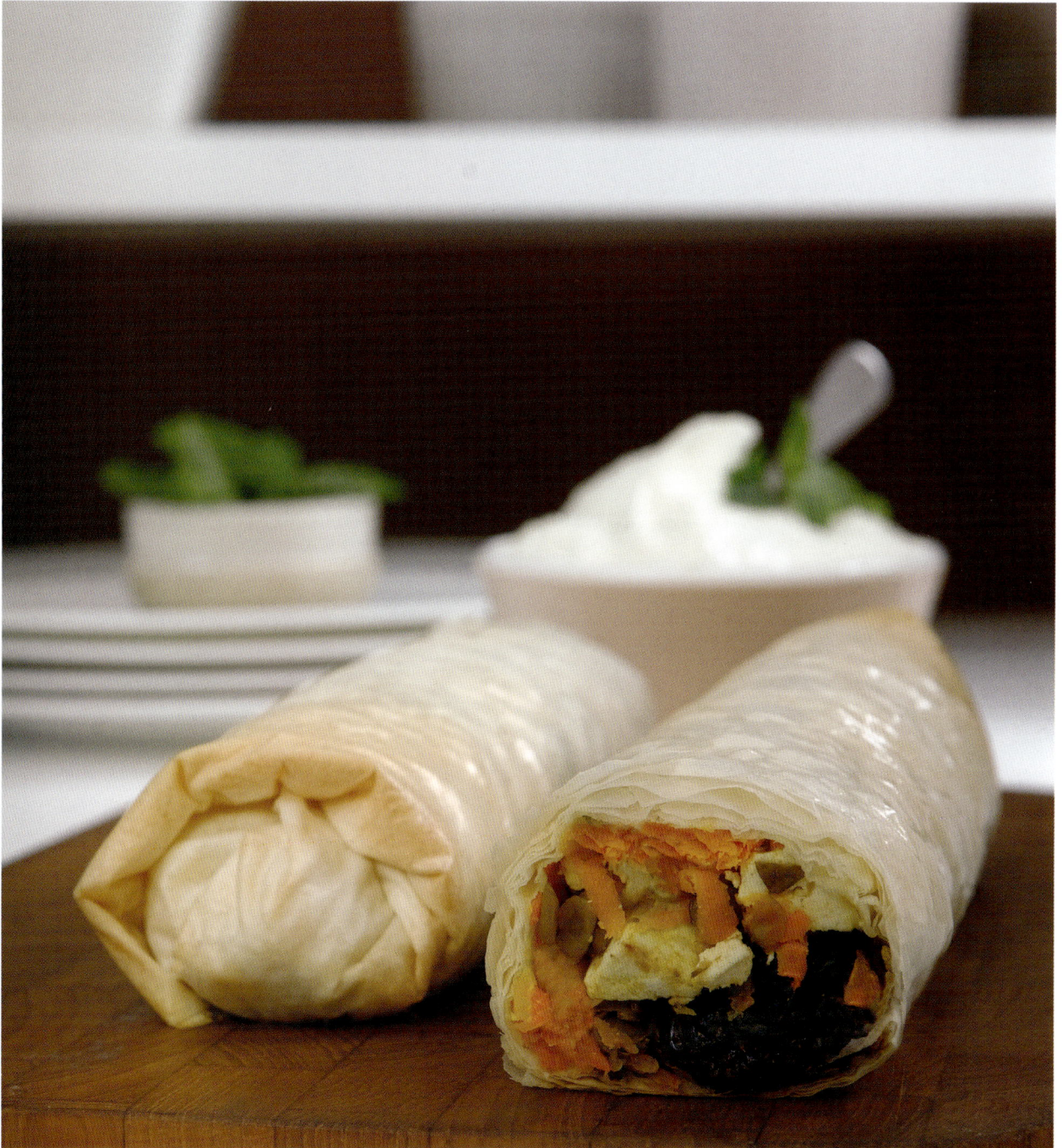

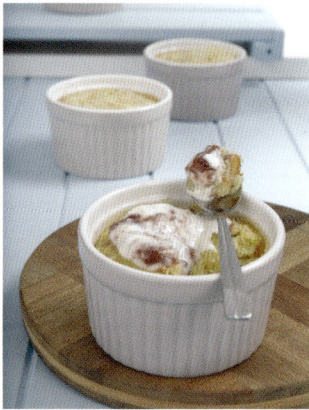
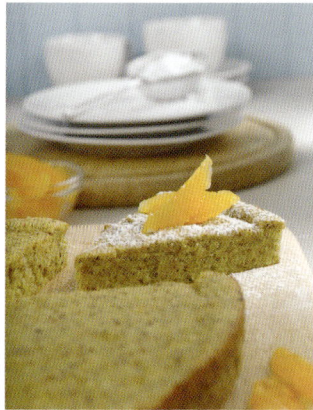
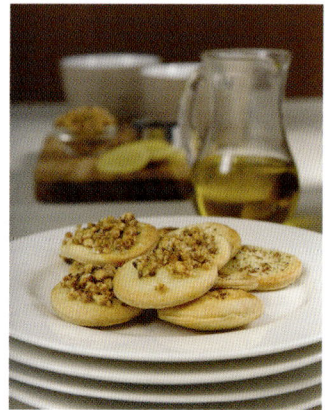

DESSERT

This was really the hardest part of the book for me as I have a devilishly sweet tooth and always have done. To create recipes that have a 'sweetness' but don't require too much sweetening was an issue.

I was determined not to use artificial sweeteners—and I haven't—so am happy with the results. While mostly based on fruit the desserts do vary. As much as I love chocolate, I have resisted any recipe for a chocolate dessert as I have just about stopped eating it. A piece of dark chocolate every now and then is good, but that is about it.

When I started this book, I talked with a foodie mate of mine in the health food area and asked her about using artificial additives. She advised that you are better not to have them. I now rarely crave for sweet things as I used to and a piece of fruit seems to suffice. Every now and then I backslide but these 'episodes' are becoming less frequent as I proceed on this wonderful way of eating sensibly and nutritiously.

Apple Jelly, Mixed Berries and Low-fat Strawberry Yoghurt

Preparation time: 5 minutes
Refrigeration time: 2 hours
Serves: 4

500ml (2 cups) natural, low-GI apple juice
1 x 7g sachet gelatine
200g strawberries, hulled and halved
60g blueberries
200g low-fat/no-fat strawberry yoghurt

1. Make the jelly by bringing 125 ml (½ cup) juice to the boil. Remove from heat and stir in the gelatine until dissolved. Pour remaining 375 ml (1½ cups) apple juice into a glass bowl and stir in the dissolved gelatine. Stir well, cool for a couple of minutes and refrigerate to set for 2 hours.
2. Combine the strawberries and blueberries.
3. When jelly is set, spoon 100g into serving glasses or bowls, top with equal amount of berries and spoon over the yoghurt.

Nutritional information: amounts per serve	
Energy (kJ)	480
Protein (g)	5
Total Fat (g)	0.2
Saturated Fat (g)	0.05
Total Carbohydrate (g)	22
Sugars (g)	22
Fibre (g)	1.3
Sodium (mg)	50
G.I.	low

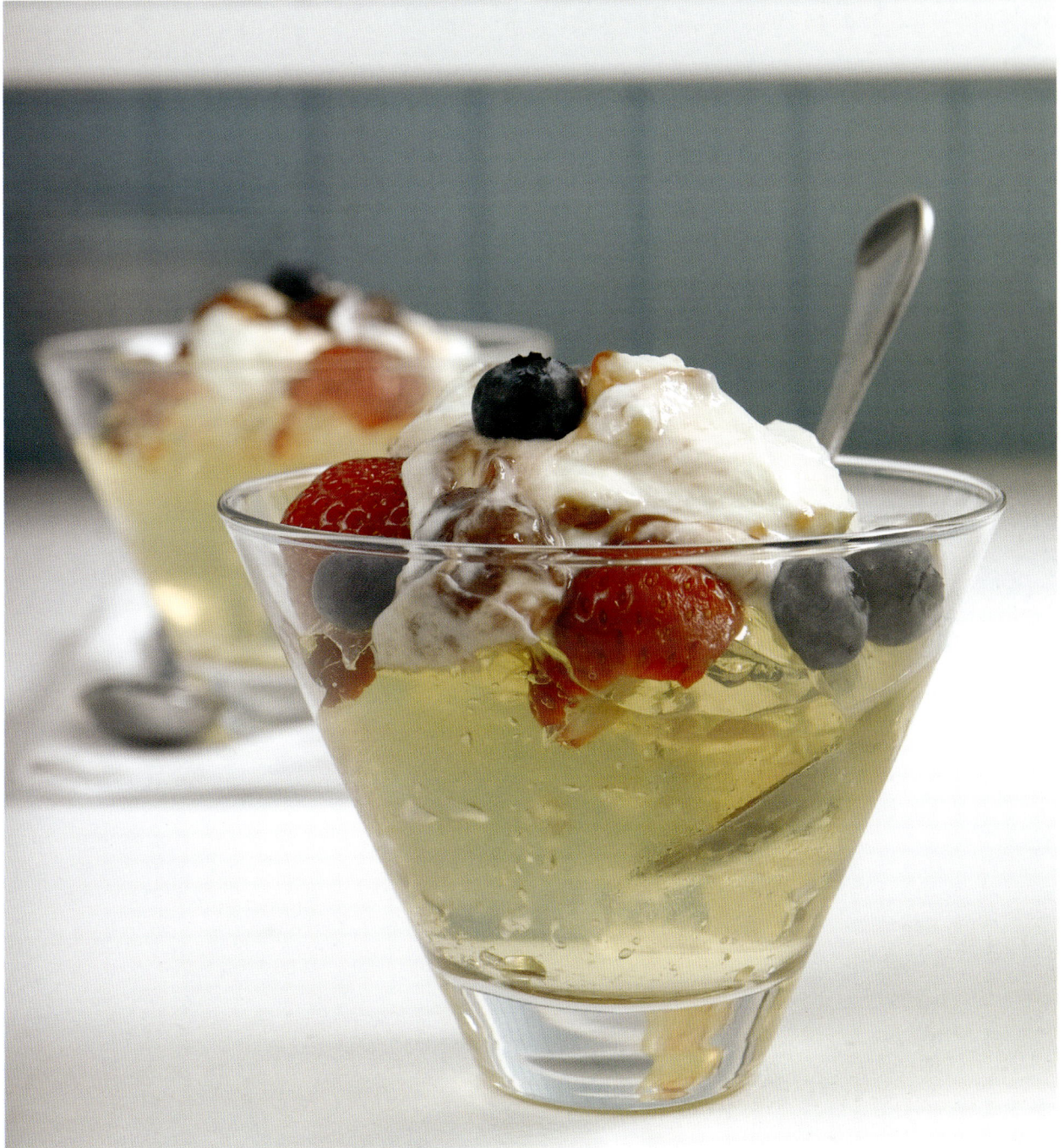

Brulèed Prune, Orange and Brandy Creams

The basis of this recipe comes from a wonderful American book called *Eating for Diabetes* by Jane Frank. I have adjusted it for my taste … and yours I hope!

Preparation time: 25 minutes (excluding overnight setting)
Serves: 6

2 cups seeded prunes
¼ cup fresh orange juice
¼ cup water
1½ cups low-fat/no-fat natural yoghurt
1 tablespoon brandy
2 tablespoons raw sugar

1. Simmer the prunes in the orange juice and water until they start to break down: around 5–7 minutes. Cool and puree. When cold, mix with the yoghurt and brandy and spoon into 6 ramekins. Refrigerate for 6 hours or overnight.
2. When ready to serve, heat the grill to as high as possible and sprinkle over equal amounts of sugar. You need to lightly coat the top with sugar, not saturate it. Place under the griller to melt and set the sugar. Let cool and serve.

This dessert is high in carbohydrates and should be balanced out with a main course that is not.

Serve with a 'meat and three vegetable meal' or a good, light salad that combines a small amount of protein with the salad ingredients.

Nutritional information: amounts per serve	
Energy (kJ)	780
Protein (g)	5
Total Fat (g)	0.4
Saturated Fat (g)	0.1
Total Carbohydrate (g)	35
Sugars (g)	28
Fibre (g)	5
Sodium (mg)	50
G.I.	low

Date and Mixed Fruit Cake

Preparation time: 15 minutes
Cooking time: 60–90 minutes
Makes: 20 slices

200g mixed fruit
275g preserved dates, chopped
440g tinned fruit salad in juice
1 cup fruit juice (I use natural, non-filtered apple juice)
½ teaspoon bicarbonate of soda
2 cups self-raising flour

1. Pre-heat oven to 180°C (fan-forced 160°C). Boil the fruit, dates, fruit salad and juice together for 10 minutes. Allow to cool for 5 minutes.
2. Mix in the bicarb and flour.
3. Turn into a lightly spray oiled cake tin and cook until done, around 1–1½ hours depending on the tin you use. See note below.

I use a 20cm square x 7cm deep tin and it cooks to a lovely, rich, moist cake that lasts for up to 14 days in an airtight container in the refrigerator.

Nutritional information: amounts per serve	
Energy (kJ)	550
Protein (g)	2
Total Fat (g)	0.5
Saturated Fat (g)	0.05
Total Carbohydrate (g)	30
Sugars (g)	19
Fibre (g)	3
Sodium (mg)	140
G.I.	low

Coconut Citrus Pudding

Preparation time: 10 minutes
Cooking time: 40 minutes
Serves: 8

4 eggs
¾ cup honey
¼ cup vegetable oil
125g almonds, chopped
1 cup (70g) coconut, desiccated
finely grated zest of 1 orange and 1 lemon
½ cup fresh orange juice
½ cup fresh lemon juice
½ cup skim milk
½ cup plain flour, sifted with 1 teaspoon baking powder
spray canola oil

1. Pre-heat oven to 180°C (fan-forced 160°C). Put all ingredients into a food processor, except for the spray canola oil, and blend for at least 1 minute.
2. Pour into a deep pie dish that has been lightly sprayed with oil.
3. Cook for 30–40 minutes or until set and golden brown. Cool and serve with flavoured yoghurt of your choice.

This cooks in 30 minutes and I leave them to cool before easing them out of the bowl. I then slice the wedges to serve 8 and serve them with the yoghurt. This is a very intense pudding, dense but delicious.

I also make this using four individual pie dishes. I use Chinese bowls and divide the mixture evenly into the four lightly oiled containers.

Nutritional information: amounts per serve	
Energy (kJ)	1740
Protein (g)	9
Total Fat (g)	25
Saturated Fat (g)	7
Total Carbohydrate (g)	39
Sugars (g)	33
Fibre (g)	3
Sodium (mg)	225
G.I.	low

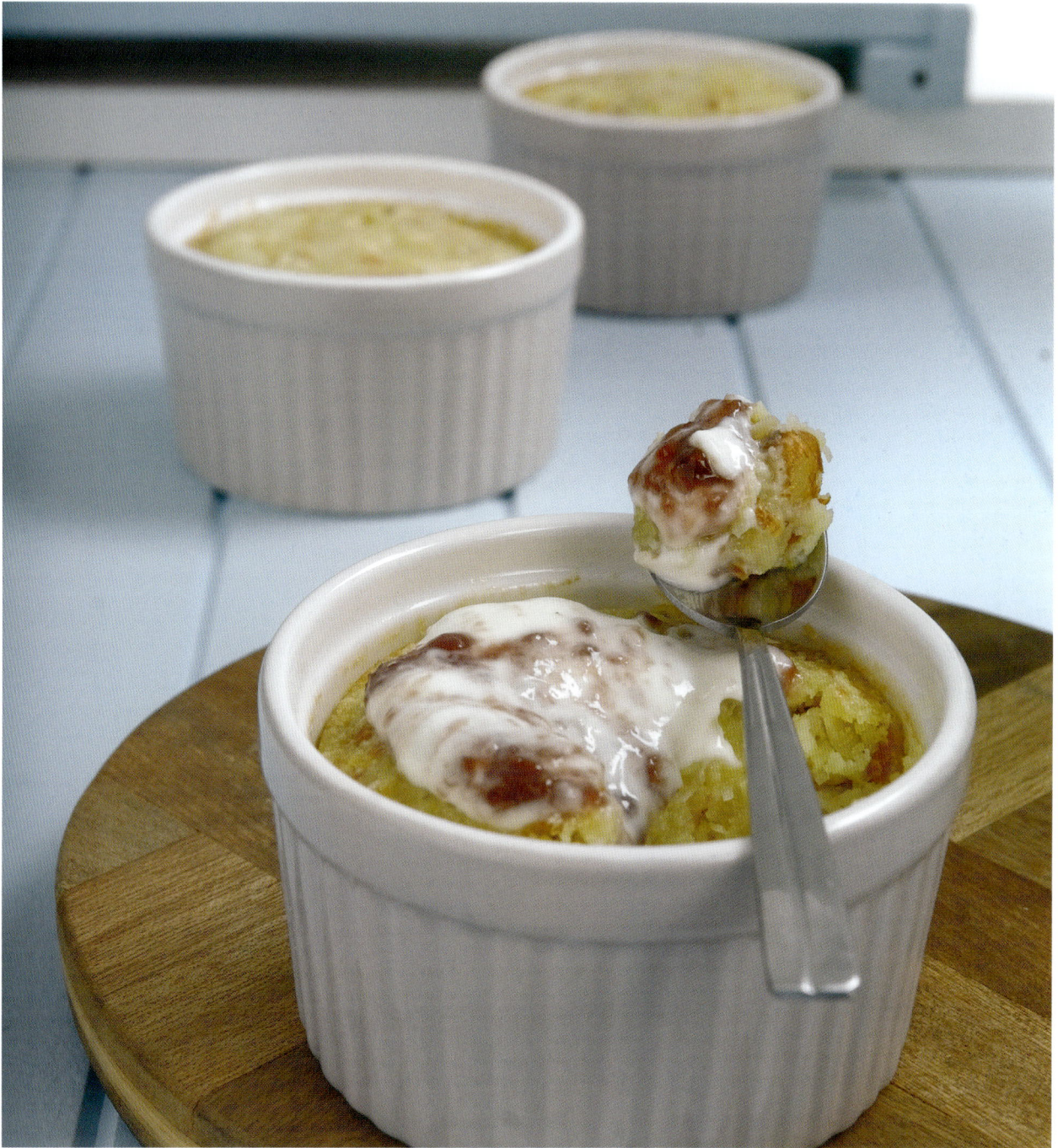

Glazed Apple Flan

Preparation time: 25 minutes
Freezer/refrigerator time: 35 minutes
Cooking time: 50 minutes
Serves: 8

1 batch olive oil pastry (see Basics page 20)
1 egg white
2 green apples
1 orange zest, finely grated and juice of half orange
1 teaspoon nutmeg, grated
2 tablespoons no-cane-sugar raspberry preserve
1 tablespoon water

Nutritional information: amounts per serve	
Energy (kJ)	840
Protein (g)	4
Total Fat (g)	8
Saturated Fat (g)	1
Total Carbohydrate (g)	28
Sugars (g)	9.5
Fibre (g)	2
Sodium (mg)	10
G.I.	medium

1. I use ¾ of this amount of pastry for a 24cm diameter x 2cm deep loose-based tart or quiche tin. Roll the pastry out between two pieces of cling wrap to about ½cm thick and line the tart/quiche tin. Trim and put in the freezer for 25 minutes. Remove and refrigerate for 10 minutes.
2. Preheat oven to 200°C (fan-forced 180°C). Take the raw pastry case from the refrigerator, prick using a fork and bake for 10 minutes. Lift from the oven and brush with some lightly beaten egg white. Let sit for a few minutes while you prepare the apples.
3. Core and halve the apples, from stem to base. Cut into half-moon slices making sure the apple half stays in place and the apple slices sit tightly together. Place in bowl and sprinkle over the orange zest and orange juice. Let sit for 2 minutes then fan the drained, sliced apples around the partially cooked pastry base. Do this in a circular movement starting with the outside first and working in the centre. You 'flatten' the sliced apple halves as you fan them. Make sure the apples are well drained and all the zest is on top of the sliced apples.
4. Cook in the oven for 35–40 minutes or until the apples are breaking down.
5. Remove and cool for 3 minutes then sprinkle with the nutmeg. Melt the preserve and water in microwave for 30 seconds, brush over the top of the apples and put back into the oven for 10 minutes. Lift from the oven and cool before removing the base and slicing. Serve with low-fat vanilla ice-cream. (Ice-cream not included in the nutritional analysis.)

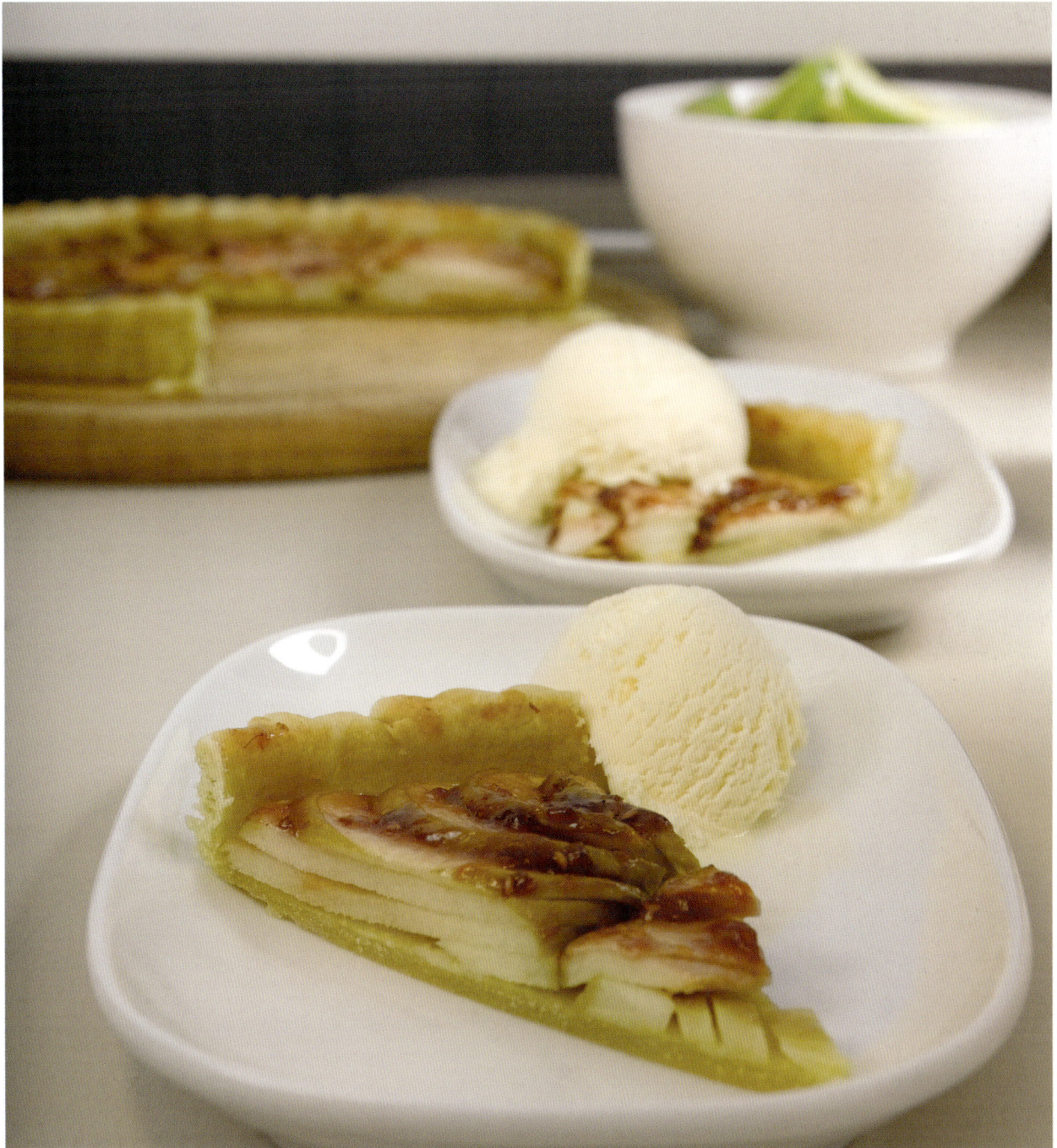

Orange and Hazelnut Cake

Preparation time: 60 minutes
Cooking time: 60–70 minutes
Makes: 10 serves

2 medium oranges, raw weight 400g
1 cinnamon curl
250g hazelnut meal
4 eggs white and 2 whole eggs
120g spelt flour
¼ cup yellow polenta
½ cup honey, warmed (in microwave) for easy pouring
1 teaspoon baking powder
1 teaspoon nutmeg, grated
2 oranges cut into skinless segments for garnish

Nutritional information: amounts per serve	
Energy (kJ)	1330
Protein (g)	9
Total Fat (g)	17
Saturated Fat (g)	1
Total Carbohydrate (g)	33
Sugars (g)	21
Fibre (g)	5
Sodium (mg)	110
G.I.	low

1. Cover the two oranges with water and bring to the boil. Break the cinnamon curl over the top, drop in, reduce to a simmer and cook for 60 minutes. When done, remove from the heat and lift out the oranges to cool. Keep the cooking liquid to use later or reduce to a syrup to spoon over the cake.
2. Line 2 x 21cm non-stick, round sponge cake tins with baking paper.
3. Preheat oven to 170ºC (fan-forced 160ºC). Break the cooked oranges open, remove seeds and drop into the food processor bowl. Add the hazelnut meal, egg white and eggs.
4. Start the processor and feed the flour, polenta, honey, baking powder and nutmeg through the shute. When combined well, pour equal amounts into each of the tins. Cook at 170ºC for 45–60 minutes or until an inserted skewer comes out clean.
5. Let the cakes cool in their tins for 10 minutes and remove to cool further. Serve with the orange segments and a sprinkle of icing sugar (optional).

This is a solid cake that does not rise very much and, when cooling, will set well. It stores well for a week in an airtight container. You will get 10 good-sized wedges from these cakes.

Spelt is an excellent flour as it reacts well in cooking and has great fibre. The polenta gives a texture I like. You can use almond meal instead of hazelnuts.

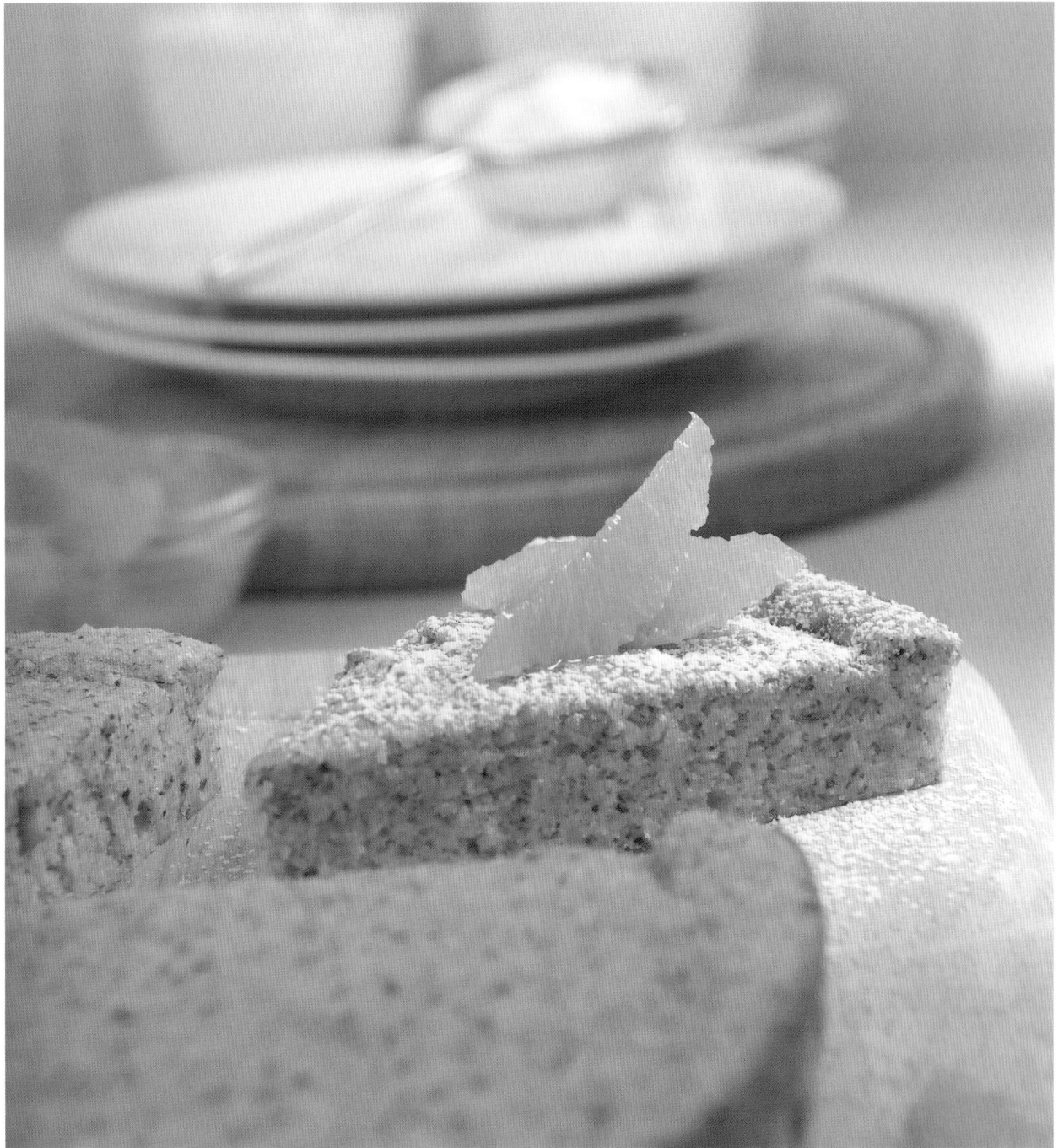

Rich Fruit Bread and Custard Pudding

Preparation time: 10 minutes
Cooking time: 50–60 minutes
Serves: 4

4 slices fruit bread
2 tablespoons no-cane-sugar-added fruit preserves
3 large eggs (67g each)
500 ml (2 cups) skim milk
½ teaspoon vanilla extract
½ teaspoon powdered cinnamon
spray canola oil

1. Preheat oven to 180°C (fan-forced 160°C). Spread 2 slices of bread with the preserve and top with the other slices to make sandwiches. Cut into triangles.
2. Beat the eggs, milk, vanilla and cinnamon until well combined.
3. Spray a baking dish with a little oil. Pack in sandwich triangles and slowly pour in the egg mixture.
4. Put the baking dish into a deeper baking dish and fill the bottom dish with cold water to be halfway up the side of the first baking dish (a bain-marie). Put into oven to cook for 50–60 minutes or until the egg mixture has set. Serve warm.

Nutritional information: amounts per serve	
Energy (kJ)	1100
Protein (g)	14
Total Fat (g)	7
Saturated Fat (g)	2
Total Carbohydrate (g)	36
Sugars (g)	23
Fibre (g)	3
Sodium (mg)	210
G.I.	low

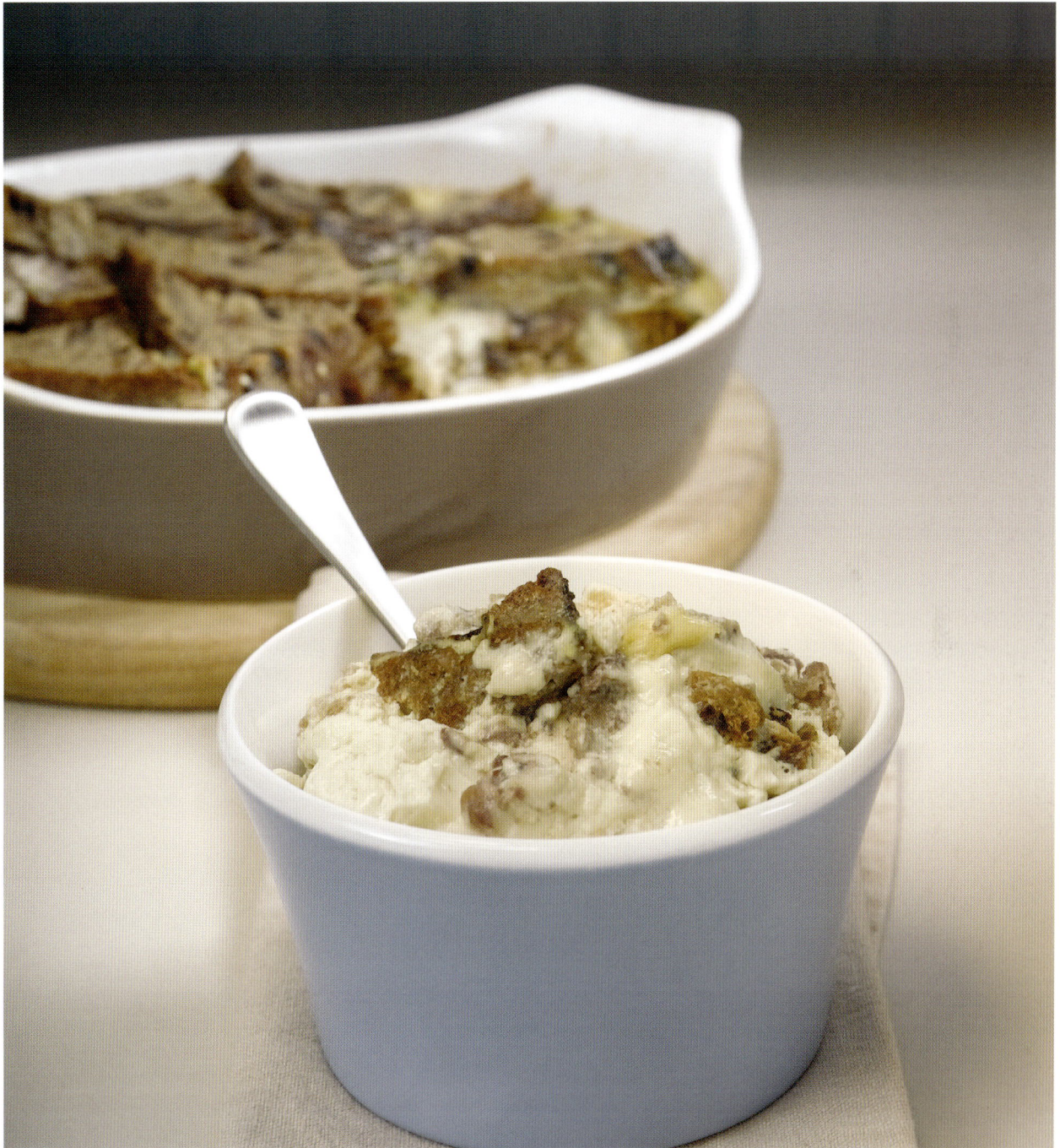

Orange Mango Flummery with Mango and Almonds

Preparation time: 20 minutes
Refrigeration time: 2 hours
Serves: 4 big serves

1 x 9g sachet orange mango light jelly
250 ml (1 cup) boiling water
250 ml (1 cup) cold water
2 egg whites
185 ml (¾ cup approximately) light and creamy evaporated milk, put in the freezer for 1 hour before use
1 cup sliced mango, canned and drained
½ cup almond slivers, toasted

Nutritional information: amounts per serve	
Energy (kJ)	820
Protein (g)	12
Total Fat (g)	10
Saturated Fat (g)	1.1
Total Carbohydrate (g)	13.5
Sugars (g)	13
Fibre (g)	2.2
Sodium (mg)	230
G.I.	low

1. Tip the jelly into a large bowl and stir in 250ml boiling water. Stir well to dissolve the powder. Pour in the cold water and stir. Cool for a couple of minutes then refrigerate for about an hour.
2. When the jelly is starting to set you'll notice it around the edges of the bowl. The larger the bowl the quicker it will set. Whisk the egg whites with an electric beater. Once soft peaks are formed, refrigerate. Whisk the slightly frozen milk in a chilled bowl (from the freezer). It will become thick but not like whipped cream.
3. Put the jelly, egg whites and milk on the bench. Beat the jelly with the electric beaters for 20 seconds, lower the beaters into the milk and pour in the jelly with the beater on slow. Ensure the mixture is well combined. Fold in the egg whites and refrigerate covered for 45–60 minutes.
4. Serve decorated with equal amounts of mango slices and sprinkled with the almonds.

This tangy, fluffy dessert is hard to stop eating. It is a special time dessert and you will not be able to keep your family from it. It can be tricky to bring all the ingredients to just their right consistency, but do persevere as the results are really worth it.

SNACKS AND SOUPS

Snacking was a part of my life. What I snacked on was the problem. I was so overweight simply because I ate all the time. Today, when I am working, I still feel the urge for a snack around the 4.00pm mark.

I have designed recipes that make for snacks and soups that are always there. The soups can be used as a more substantial snack or even turned into a savoury smoothie. During summer this is great poured onto ice and consumed.

How often do your friends drop around for a drink or 'a cuppa' in the afternoon? At my house this often occurs, so it's nice to have something more interesting than a bag of potato crisps and store-purchased dips.

Here are some solutions to that snack attack.

Black Eye Bean Paste

Preparation time: 10 minutes
Cooking time: 50–60 minutes
Makes: 2–3 cups or 500g–750g

250g soaked black eye beans
4 cloves garlic, poached
2 tablespoons lime juice
1 teaspoon powdered cumin
1 teaspoon powdered nutmeg
½ teaspoon ground white pepper
¼ teaspoon powdered chilli
¼ teaspoon salt
1 tablespoon canola oil
1 tablespoon parsley, chopped

1. Cook the beans at a simmer until they start to break down. Strain and save a cup of the cooking liquid.
2. Put all the ingredients, except the oil and parsley, into a processor and work to a paste. You may need to add some cooking liquid to give the paste the consistency you like, but it should be smooth and creamy. It will have black specks through it from the beans.
3. Spoon or lift the paste into a bowl and smooth it over the top with a knife.
4. Spoon over the olive oil and sprinkle with parsley. Serve with good rye, rye and linseed or similar bread.

I like to toast the bread before I use it. I have found, however, that good quality, healthy breads stay fresh longer, so this delicious filling spreads on more easily. To make this into a lunch meal you can top with tomato, rocket and squeeze lemon juice all over.

This recipe may look high in sodium, but that is for the whole lot. When you look at how much you use in a serve, it is quite reasonable.

Nutritional information: amounts per serve: standard serve size 29g	
Energy (kJ)	155
Protein (g)	1.5
Total Fat (g)	1.7
Saturated Fat (g)	0.1
Total Carbohydrate (g)	3
Sugars (g)	0.5
Fibre (g)	1.5
Sodium (mg)	120
G.I.	low

Chocolate, Banana and Kiwi Fruit Smoothie

Preparation time: 5 minutes
Makes: 3 good-sized drinks

100g 97% fat-free chocolate swirl ice-cream
150g very ripe Cavendish bananas
75g kiwi fruit, peeled
1 tablespoon lemon juice
2 cups skim milk
½ teaspoon powdered cinnamon

Put all ingredients, except the cinnamon, into a blender and work until combined. Pour and sprinkle with cinnamon.

This is a great afternoon snack. When I am working in the office, I get so hungry around 4.00pm and make this drink to see me through to dinner. It is also great to blend in 5–6 ice cubes during the hot sub-tropical weather I get where I live.

Nutritional information: amounts per serve	
Energy (kJ)	730
Protein (g)	9
Total Fat (g)	1.5
Saturated Fat (g)	0.9
Total Carbohydrate (g)	30
Sugars (g)	27
Fibre (g)	33
Sodium (mg)	100
G.I.	low

Cinnamon Lemongrass Tea

Preparation time: 15 minutes
Serves: 4 cups

3 x 8cm long cinnamon quills
1 small lemon, cut in halves
6 x 20cm long pieces green lemongrass leaves
4 cups boiling water

1. Break the cinnamon quills in half and drop into a teapot with the lemon halves.
2. Crush the lemongrass leaves and add to the other ingredients. Top with boiling water and leave to steep or infuse for 10 minutes.
3. Strain and drink hot, warm or at room temperature.

This is really refreshing as a hot drink and is good chilled too. Strain it into a glass container before chilling. Don't keep much longer than a day as the aroma that makes it so attractive slowly dissipates when storing. I pour it over ice with some lemon slices in summer for a long drink any time of day.

Cinnamon quills or sticks are the best to use. I have loved that wonderfully exotic aroma since I was a kid.

Nutritional information: amounts per serve	
Energy (kJ)	33
Protein (g)	0.1
Total Fat (g)	0.1
Saturated Fat (g)	0
Total Carbohydrate (g)	2
Sugars (g)	0.5
Fibre (g)	1
Sodium (mg)	1
G.I.	n/a

Cinnamon Zucchini Bread

Preparation time: 15 minutes
Cooking time: 60 minutes
Makes: 2 loaves (slice into 40g slices to serve)

375g small zucchinis, washed, trimmed and grated
1 egg beaten with 2 egg whites and 1 tablespoon olive oil
1 tablespoon honey
1 teaspoon ground cinnamon
3 cups self-raising wholemeal flour
1 teaspoon baking powder
½ cup walnuts, crumbled
spray olive oil

1. Pre-heat oven to 170°C (fan-forced 150°C). Mix the zucchinis, eggs and oil, honey and cinnamon. Stir to combine well.
2. Fold in the flour, baking poweder and walnuts then leave to sit for 5 minutes. 3. Spray 2 bread tins (21cm long x 11cm wide and 6cm deep) with olive oil. Spoon equal amounts of the zucchini mixture into the tins and cook in the oven for 1 hour or until a skewer comes out clean.
4. Leave in tin for 10 minutes to cool and turn onto a cooking rack to cool before slicing. This will freeze very well.

This is a very good snack, relatively savoury and solid. The walnuts give it that desirable crunch and the zucchini keeps the bread moist during cooking.

You can slice it and store refrigerated in an airtight container for at least 7 days. Toast it for a variation to serve with soups or with sugar-free preserves.

Nutritional information: amounts per 40g slice	
Energy (kJ)	384
Protein (g)	3
Total Fat (g)	3.3
Saturated Fat (g)	0.5
Total Carbohydrate (g)	11.5
Sugars (g)	1.5
Fibre (g)	2.5
Sodium (mg)	140
G.I.	medium

Creamy Leek and Kumara Soup

Preparation time: 10 minutes
Cooking time: 30 minutes
Serves: 5

1½L sodium-reduced vegetable stock
200g leeks, white part only and roughly chopped
500g kumara (orange sweet potato), peeled and roughly chopped
½ teaspoon cayenne
½ cup reduced fat evaporated milk (98.5% fat-free)

1. Put the stock, leek and kumara into a suitable pot and bring to the boil then simmer for 30 minutes. When the kumara starts to break down, remove from the heat and puree in a food processor or with a hand blender.
2. Add the cayenne and evaporated milk; reheat, stirring as you do and taking care not to boil. Serve with wholemeal bread rolls or rye bread toast.

This nutritional soup is a good start to a meal or a meal on its own. To give it more body you can reduce it by simmering or you can add low-fat or no-fat natural yoghurt. The other bonus is that it can be used as a base for vegetable casseroles.

Nutritional information: amounts per serve	
Energy (kJ)	580
Protein (g)	11
Total Fat (g)	1
Saturated Fat (g)	0.2
Total Carbohydrate (g)	20
Sugars (g)	10.5
Fibre (g)	3
Sodium (mg)	800
G.I.	low

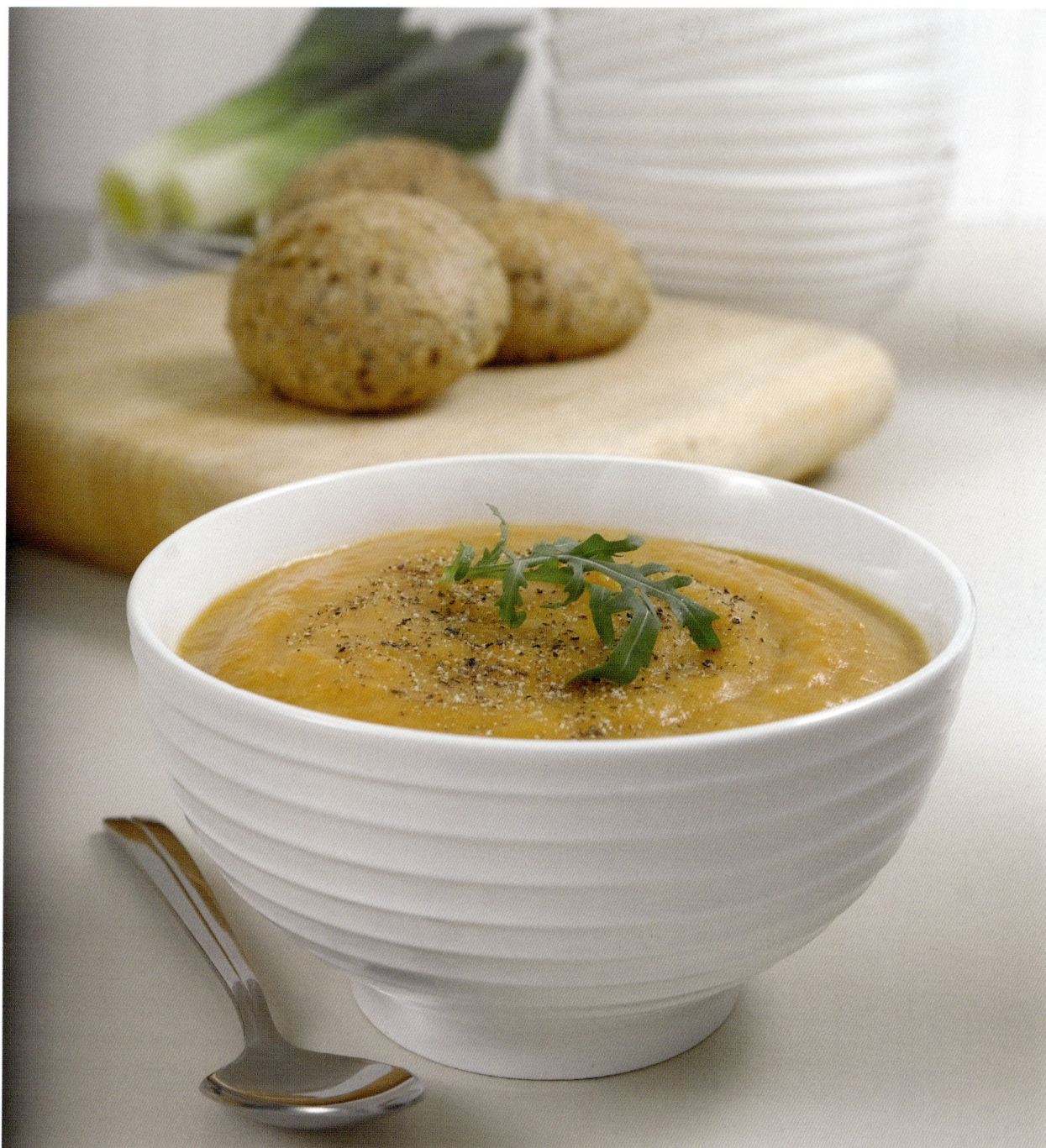

Flavoured Olive Oil Biscuits

Preparation time: 15 minutes
Cooking time: 25 minutes
Makes: 8 biscuits (or 4 x 2 per serve)

150g olive oil pastry (see Basics page 20)
1 egg white
various toppings: dukkah (see Basics page 18), sumac, flaked dried onions, etc.
spray canola oil

1. Preheat oven to 200ºC (fan-forced 180ºC). Roll the pastry to 1/2cm thick and cut into rounds using a biscuit cutter (6.5cm in diameter). Lift onto a lightly oil-sprayed oven tray that you have a duplicate of and refrigerate for 10 minutes.
2. Take the tray from the refrigerator and prick each biscuit with a fork. Cover with the identical tray and cook for 10 minutes in the oven.
3. Lift from the oven and cool for 5 minutes. Brush with the egg white and sprinkle on you toppings. I use my dukkah, the spice sumac and onion flakes. Bake for a further 10 minutes in the oven. Remove from oven, cool on a rack and serve at room temperature.

These will store in an airtight container for 5 days.

Nutritional information: amounts per serve (2 biscuits each)	
Energy (kJ)	640
Protein (g)	4
Total Fat (g)	7
Saturated Fat (g)	1
Total Carbohydrate (g)	17
Sugars (g)	1
Fibre (g)	1
Sodium (mg)	17
G.I.	medium

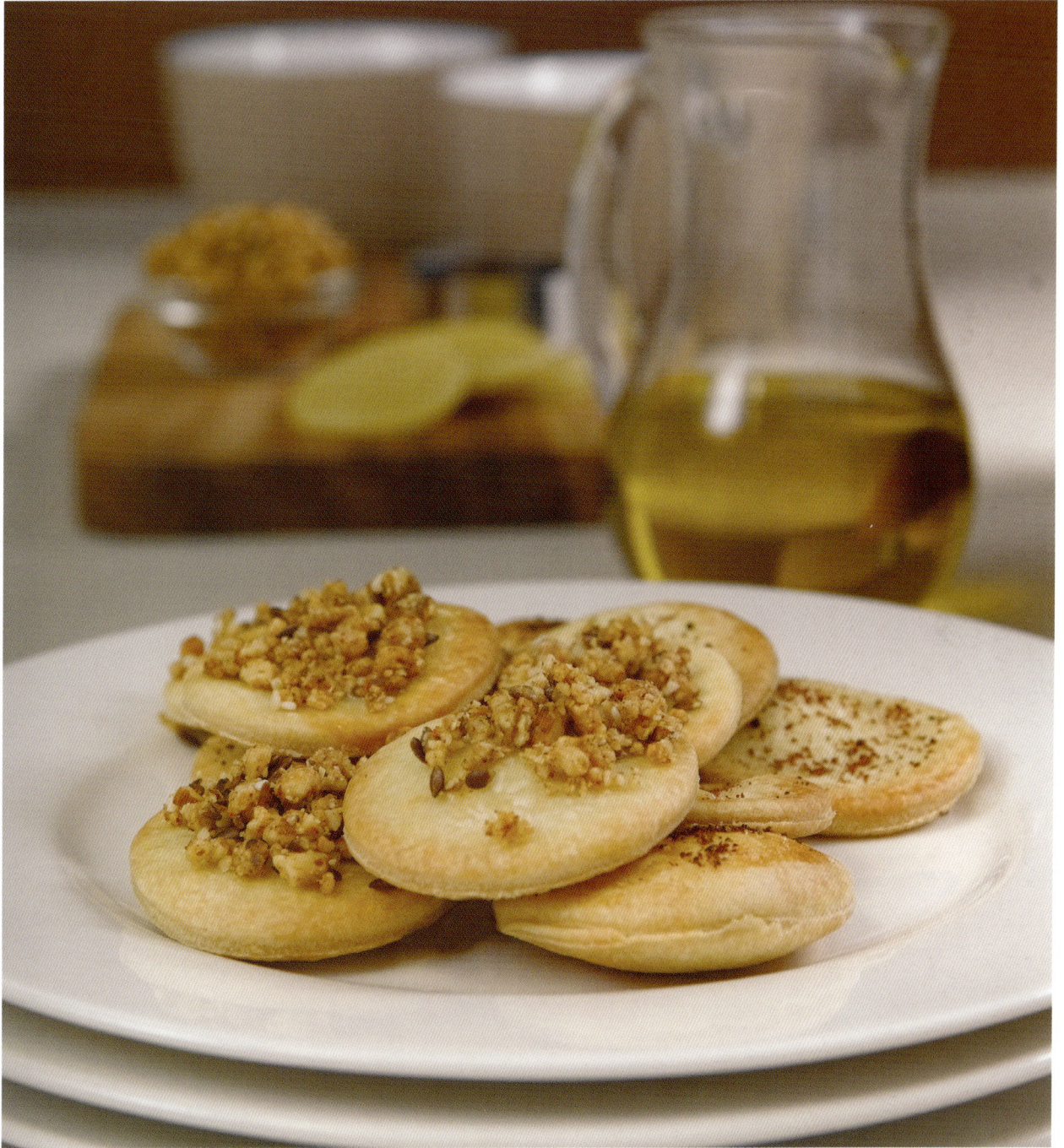

Kumara and Pink Salmon Cakes

Preparation time: 20 minutes
Cooking time: 20 minutes
Makes: 8 cakes (2 cakes per serve)

200g steamed kumara (orange sweet potato)
100g steamed potato (Pontiac or Sebago)
200g drained salmon in spring water
1 egg
2 tablespoons parsley, chopped
1 tablespoon allspice
½ teaspoon ground black pepper
4 tablespoons barley bran
organic plain flour for coating
spray canola oil for pan frying

1. Mash the kumara, potato, salmon, egg, parsley, allspice and pepper together. Gradually add the bran to take up excess moisture. You shouldn't have to use all the bran—try not to dry out the mixture.
2. Make eight even-sized patties. Dust them in flour and sit in the refrigerator until ready to use. Cook in minimum oil and serve hot or warm. Alternatively, you can spray these with a little canola oil and bake them in the oven, at 180ºC, until lightly browned and crisp. Serve hot or at room temperature.

One of the advantages of these tasty treats is that they can be transformed into a meal. I have served them with a salad for lunch, and for dinner with stewed cabbage, flavoured with a splash of red wine and caraway seeds. Good wholemeal bread rolls set both meals off beautifully.

Nutritional information: amounts for serve of 2 cakes	
Energy (kJ)	730
Protein (g)	14
Total Fat (g)	6
Saturated Fat (g)	1.5
Total Carbohydrate (g)	15
Sugars (g)	3.5
Fibre (g)	4
Sodium (mg)	81
G.I.	low

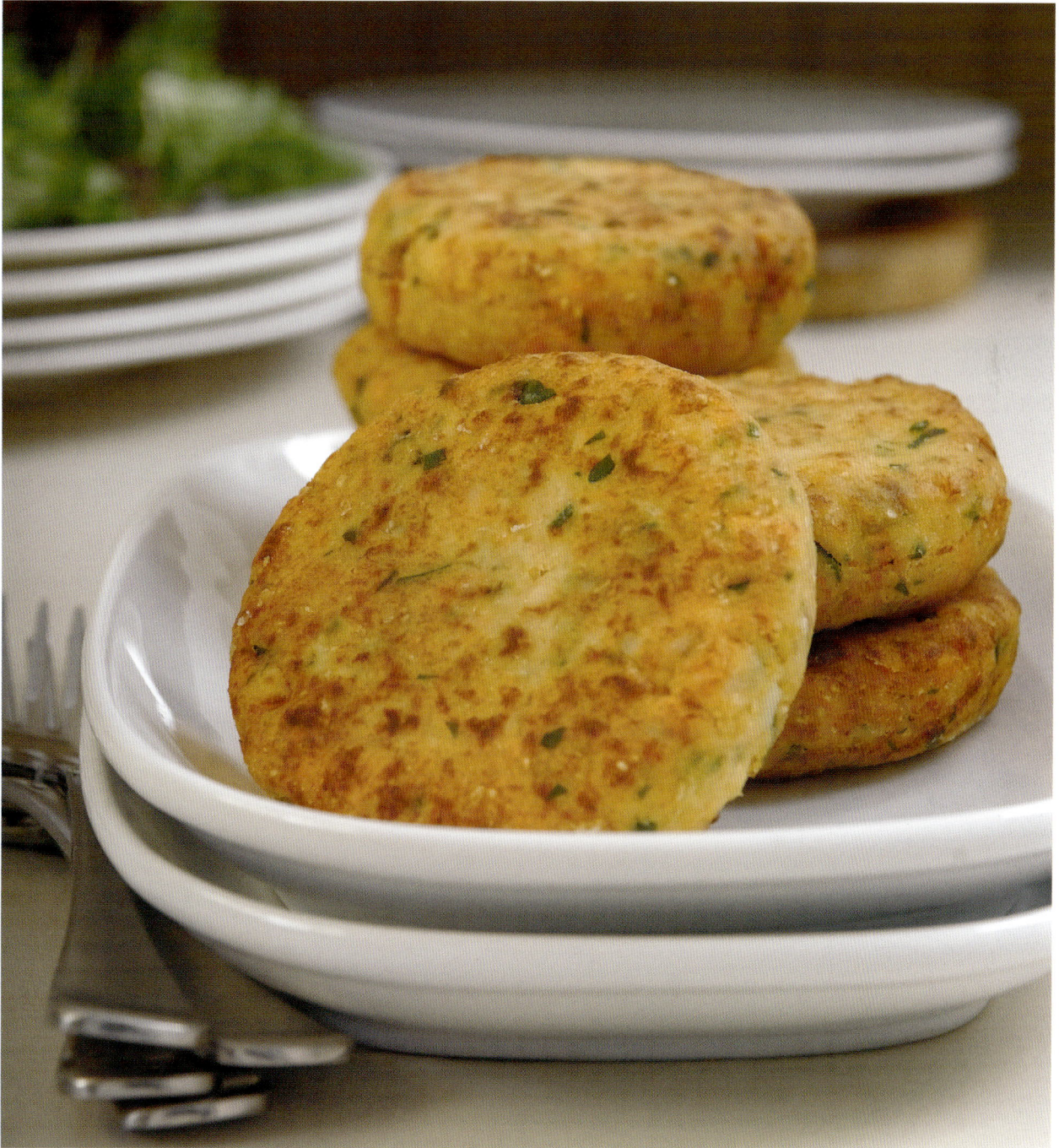

Low-fat Cheese and Olive Oil Scones

Preparation time: 10 minutes
Cooking time: 15 minutes
Makes: 12 medium-sized-scones

2 cups wholemeal self-raising flour
½ cup low-fat cottage cheese
1 tablespoon olive oil
1 cup skim milk
1 tablespoon chives, chopped
extra flour for benchwork
baking paper
extra skim milk for brushing the scones for baking

1. Pre-heat oven to 220°C (fan-forced 200°C). Make a well in the flour in a mixing bowl. Add the cheese, stir in the oil and milk gradually.
2. When roughly combined, tip onto a floured bench and work into a dough. Do not overwork. Shape into a rectangle, leaving the dough 4cm thick. Cut into even squares and place onto a baking paper-lined baking tray.
3. Brush with the extra skim milk and cook in the oven for 12–15 minutes or until risen and browned.

These fill you up and, even better, they will freeze. They are the best scones I have made for reheating in the microwave. They come out moist and stay that way. Other scones dry out and become tough.

Nutritional information: amounts per scone	
Energy (kJ)	330
Protein (g)	4
Total Fat (g)	2
Saturated Fat (g)	0.4
Total Carbohydrate (g)	10
Sugars (g)	1.5
Fibre (g)	1.6
Sodium (mg)	120
G.I.	medium

Quick Chilled Summer Vegie Soup

Preparation time: 10 minutes
chilling time: 30 minutes.
Serves: 4

600 ml (2¼ cups) tomato juice (no added sugar)
2 ripe, medium-sized tomatoes, halved, deseeded and roughly chopped
½ cup cucumber flesh, no seeds and roughly chopped
1 small red onion, peeled and roughly diced
1 medium green capsicum, deseeded and roughly diced
½ teaspoon ground ginger
½ teaspoon ground black pepper
1 tablespoon chopped parsley
ice cubes
1 cup garlic croutons (see Basics page 16)

1. Stir the juice, tomatoes, cucumber, onion, capsicum, ginger and ground black pepper together and refrigerate for at least 30 minutes.
2. To serve, stir in the parsley and spoon over 4–5 ice cubes. into four bowls. Put the croutons on the table for self service.

If you want a savoury smoothie, this is the base for one. Just put the ingredients, including some ice, in a blender and work to a smoothie consistency. Serve over ice if you like.

Nutritional information: amounts per serve	
Energy (kJ)	320
Protein (g)	3.5
Total Fat (g)	1
Saturated Fat (g)	0.1
Total Carbohydrate (g)	10
Sugars (g)	7
Fibre (g)	3
Sodium (mg)	510
G.I.	low

Soya Bean, Cinnamon and Star-Anise Soup

Preparation time: 5 minutes
Cooking time: 30 minutes
Makes: 4 big serves

3 cups soy beans, cooked and drained
1L salt-reduced chicken stock mixed with 750ml water
1 large onion, roughly chopped
3 cloves garlic, chopped
1 x 8cm-long cinnamon quill
1 star-anise
1 tablespoon curry powder
4 tablespoons creamy natural yoghurt
cracked black pepper

Nutritional information: amounts per serve	
Energy (kJ)	1070
Protein (g)	25
Total Fat (g)	11
Saturated Fat (g)	1.7
Total Carbohydrate (g)	11
Sugars (g)	7
Fibre (g)	11
Sodium (mg)	1030
G.I.	low

1. Bring the soy beans, stock, onion, cinnamon and star-anise to the boil. Reduce to simmer and cook for 30 minutes or until the beans are soft.
2. Remove the star-anise, pour the cooked contents and liquid into a food processor and puree.
3. Pour back into saucepan and add the curry powder. Bring back to a simmer and cook for 5 minutes while stirring constantly.
4. Ladle into individual soup bowls and top with a spoon of yoghurt. Sprinkle with plenty of cracked black pepper.

This is a 'substantial' soup that I serve for dinner with very good bread or wholemeal bread rolls. It is thick, will fill you up and keep you filled. Any soup you have left over will store extremely well in an airtight container in the refrigerator.

To turn this into a main course, think about adding some steamed, diced tofu to increase the protein.

If you start with dried soy beans they need to be soaked overnight and cooked. If you use salt in your cooking, add it when you puree. Salt will make the beans tough if added at the start of cooking.

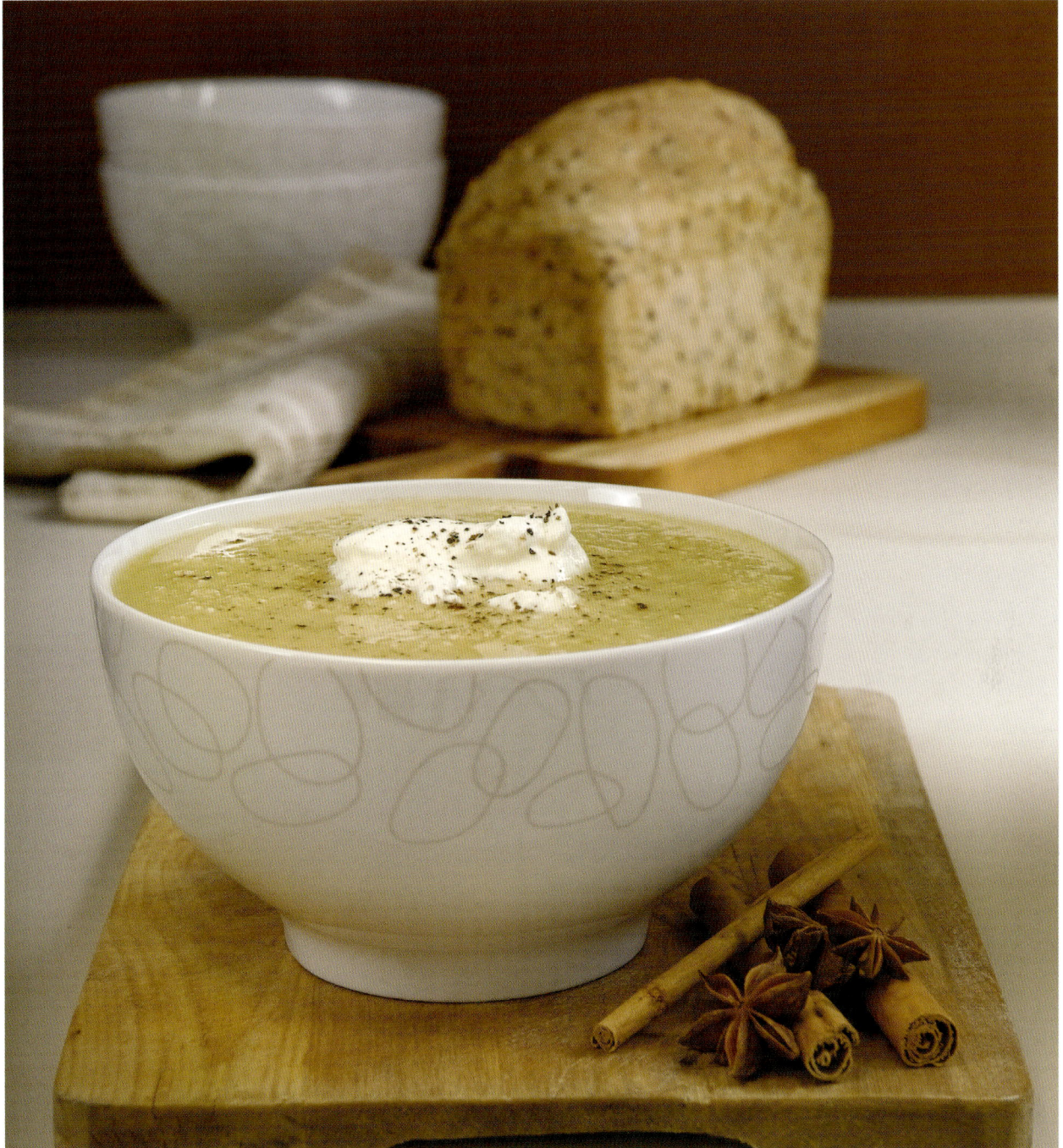

Spiced Almonds

Preparation and cooking time: 10 minutes
Makes: 6 serves

1 teaspoon coriander seeds
1 teaspoon caraway seeds
1 teaspoon dried onion
1 teaspoon dried rosemary pieces
½ teaspoon allspice
¼ teaspoon chilli powder
125g almonds (skin on)
spray olive or canola oil

1. Pound the coriander and caraway seeds using a mortar and pestle until broken down.
2. Combine them with the onion, rosemary, allspice and chilli, mix well and tip into a small non-stick frying pan.
3. Add the almonds and spray lightly with the oil. Cook over medium heat, tossing all the time. Spray again with a little oil and you will notice that the mix is sticking to the almonds. I spray mine three times with small amounts of oil.
4. After around 3–4 minutes tip them out and cool before eating. You can store them at room temperature in an airtight container, if not used all at one time.

Nutritional information: amounts for 6 serves	
Energy (kJ)	570
Protein (g)	4.5
Total Fat (g)	12.5
Saturated Fat (g)	1
Total Carbohydrate (g)	1.1
Sugars (g)	1
Fibre (g)	2
Sodium (mg)	3
G.I.	n/a

Tomato, Corn and Wholemeal Bread Slice

Preparation time: 10 minutes
Cooking time: 30–40 minutes
Cooling time: 15 minutes
Makes: 18 squares, sliced 2–3 cm thick

1 whole egg and 4 egg whites
1 cup skin milk mixed with ½ cup low sodium vegetable stock
1 cup diced 98% fat-free, semi-roasted tomatoes
1 cup corn kernels, canned or bottled
4 cups 2-day-old wholemeal bread crumbs (5 slices)
1 cup 93% fat-free cheddar-style cheese, grated
1 small green chilli, minced
1 tablespoon mixed herbs
spray canola oil

1. Pre-heat oven to 180°C (fan-forced 160°). Whisk together the eggs, egg whites, milk and stock. Stir in the tomatoes, corn and bread crumbs.
2. Fold in the cheese, chilli and herbs. Pour into a non-stick baking tray sprayed with a film of canola oil. Cook for 30–40 minutes or until an inserted skewer or knife comes out clean and the top is lightly crisped.
3. Cool on cake rack for 15 minutes before serving warm or cool to serve as a slice. To make this a more substantial meal, serve with a small green salad on the side, some tomato wedges and sprinkle with lemon juice.

I use two tins to bake this delicious savoury slice. These are 24cm square and 5cm deep. These are great to take to work: they are both delicious and portable. They can also be reheated and made crispy all over by pan-frying with spray oil in a non-stick pan.

Nutritional information: amounts per serve	
Energy (kJ)	560
Protein (g)	11
Total Fat (g)	3
Saturated Fat (g)	1
Total Carbohydrate (g)	14
Sugars (g)	3
Fibre (g)	3
Sodium (mg)	330
G.I.	low

Spicy Cannellini Hummus and Bruschetta

Preparation time: 10 minutes
Cooking time: 5 minutes
Makes: 4 serves

450g drained, cooked cannellini beans, reserve some liquid
4 cloves garlic, poached
2 tablespoons lime juice
1 teaspoon powdered cumin
1 teaspoon powdered nutmeg
½ teaspoon ground white pepper
¼ teaspoon powdered chilli
2 tablespoons olive oil
6 x 50g slices rye or wholemeal bread
2 cups trimmed rocket leaves or mixed lettuce leaves

1. Puree all ingredients except for the oil, bread and rocket in a processor and work to a paste, adding reserved bean liquid to make a smooth paste. Remove from processor.
2. Brush oil onto the bread and lightly grill. Spread 60g of the bean hummus onto the grilled bread, top with rocket leaves and serve.

If you use regular wholemeal slices, you may want to use less hummus than suggested on each slice. Regular slices are best cut into two triangles and offered as 3 triangles per serve. Any leftover hummus can be stored in an airtight container and refrigerated for up to a week.

Nutritional information: amounts per serve	
Energy (kJ)	1480
Protein (g)	18
Total Fat (g)	9
Saturated Fat (g)	1.2
Total Carbohydrate (g)	45
Sugars (g)	3
Fibre (g)	14
Sodium (mg)	345
G.I.	low

Pete's Points

These are some of the things I noticed or jotted down as I was writing the book—and since being diagnosed with Type 2 diabetes. They come in no order of importance but as they happened!

- Join Diabetes Australia immediately and talk with them whenever you need to. They are a wonderful group of people who are there to help.
- Canned fruits are fine. Use the ones that are prepared in juice, not syrup.
- Buy fresh when you can, but there is nothing wrong with frozen vegetables provided they are thawed properly.
- Snacks: always have them on hand. I always have almonds and hazelnuts when I feel the need for a quick nibble. I also love them with no-fat or low-fat flavoured yoghurt. They give a crunch and flavour that makes the yoghurt's consistency more attractive.
- Low GI breads like the Burgen range are fantastic. They are delicious, filling and nutritious. I particularly like the Rye, the Soy-Lin and, for a fruit bread, you can't go past their Fruit and Muesli.
- You must look after your feet. Going for a foot massage or other treatment is not a luxury, but a pampering you must have on a regular basis. I rub moisturiser into my feet regularly, though never between the toes.
- Explore the use of herbs and spices. They really add flavour and taste to some of the low-fat food I now eat. These foods may be extremely good for me but can lack flavour.
- Massel stocks: these Aussie stocks are very good. I buy the cubes, which take less space in my larder (pantry/cupboard).
- Oils: look into them and find the best ones for you. Always have spray oil on hand as it limits the amount you use and a fine film of oil in non-stick cookware is enough.
- Have good quality, non-stick cookware. It is invaluable.

- Make sure you have good shoes—that give support where it is needed—to exercise in: they are crucial.
- If you get bored walking, or whichever way you exercise, walk with friends, buy a good portable music player with enthusiastic, brisk music or listen to the radio as you walk. Use anything that makes you do it!

- Books you must have are
  - *The New Glucose Revolution* by Prof. Jennie Brand-Miller and Kaye Foster-Powell. This dynamic team has published many books about the Glycemic Index. Their writing is easy to follow, well explained and you feel empathy from them: and no put-downs. They also have a book called *GI Values 2005,* which is a pocket book to take shopping with you.
  - Anything by Pamela Clark from the *Australian Women's Weekly* on weight loss. Her books and words are inspirational as she has shed so much weight. One of my endeavours was to lose as much weight as I could. Pamela has done it well given she has to work around food all day and go out to represent her magazine regularly. Her book, *The Magazine Editors' Diet,* and subsequent books are excellent.
  - Looking at books I had only ever glanced at, I rediscovered a world of food that I had known about and promptly forgotten (I studied food in depth at catering college in 1970). I had listened to the brilliance of people such as Catherine Saxelby, but not really listened because they asked me to re-think my gluttonous eating habits. Catherine's *Everyday Diet Secrets* is a pocket book that reinforces your resolve.
- Buy the *Healthy Shopping Guide* by Diabetes Australia for invaluable advice.

How to Make Sense of Food Labels

by Catherine Saxelby

When you scan the back of the pack at your local shop, do you ask questions like these?
- What is food acid (330)?
- Or vegetable gum (415)?
- If it says 'light' does that mean it's low in fat?

Follow these five easy steps to help you interpret what that fine print really means.

STEP 1: Check the Ingredient List

What's really in this food? Let's check the Ingredient List on the back of the pack.

All ingredients must be stated in order of decreasing weight. The first is the largest, followed by the second, the third, and so on.

In these labels fat can appear as:
- vegetable oil (in snack foods and sauces)
- vegetable shortening (in muffins and cakes)
- ghee
- lard
- suet
- coconut cream
- copha

While sugar can be derived from:
- sucrose (chemical name) as in cane sugar
- fructose (fruit sugar) as in corn syrup
- glucose
- extrose (another name for glucose)
- golden syrup
- treacle
- concentrated pear juice/syrup

What can we tell from this sample food label for French salad dressing?
The first thing we see is that the main Ingredient, *sunflower oil*, makes up 60 per cent of the dressing. Then *water* and *vinegar* are there in smaller proportions with *salt, sugar, food acid, gum, spice, herbs, garlic, colour* and *antioxidant* present only in minute amounts (similar to 'a pinch' in a recipe).

If some form of sugar appears as one of the first three ingredients, the food is generally **high in added sugar**.

What's a characterising ingredient?

A characterising ingredient is one which gives the food its character. For example strawberries are the characterising ingredient of strawberry jam. While the percentage of the key ingredient in a product must be shown, it will not necessarily be the main ingredient in terms of weight.

In this dressing, the characterising ingredients are oil (which is 60 per cent of the dressing), vinegar (8 per cent) with garlic (1 per cent) giving it its flavour.

> **Sample food label**
>
> French salad dressing with garlic
> sunflower oil (60%),
> water, vinegar (8%),
> salt, sugar, food acid (330),
> vegetable gum (415),
> spice, herbs, garlic (1%),
> colour (102),
> antioxidant (320)

STEP 2: Checking the additives

Additives must be shown on the ingredient list by their functional name. For example, *food acid*, and this must be followed by either their chemical name, in this case (citric acid), or by their code number (330). This numbering system has been used in Europe for many years and you will see imported foods with the same code number preceded by the letter 'E'.

All food additives must have a specific use and must have been assessed and approved by the Food Standards Australia New Zealand (FSANZ). They must be used in the lowest possible quantity to achieve their purpose, consistent with good manufacturing practice.

Back to our salad dressing! There are four additives listed on the label:
Food acid (330) is citric acid, which adds a pleasant tang (like lemon juice).
Vegetable gum (415) is xanthan gum, a common food gum that thickens the dressing.
Colour (102) is tartrazine, which gives a golden hue to the dressing.
Antioxidant (320) is BHA (butylated hydroxy anisole), which prevents the dressing from deteriorating before its use-by-date. Remember, the dressing is not refrigerated so needs something to stop it going off.

If you would like to see the whole list of approved additives Catherine Saxelby's pocket guide *Foodwatch A to Z* puts all the information at your fingertips. It lists all the additives and their numbers as well as explaining technical terms you might see on food packs such as GI, MSG or Halal.
Find it at good bookshops or buy it online at:
http://www.foodwatch.com.au

STEP 3: Checking the Nutrition Information Panel

Nutrition figures are presented in a standard table format on most food labels. This shows the quantities per serve and per 100g of the food or 100mL if liquid.

Sample Nutrition Information Panel		
Servings per pack: 14 Serving size: 1tbsp (20ml)	Per 20ml tbsp	Per 100ml
Energy	430kJ 103Cal	2140kJ 510Cal
Protein	0.1g	0.3g
Fat, total	11g	55g
Saturated	2g	10g
Carbohydrate, total	0.1g	1g
sugars	0.1g	1g
Dietary fibre	0g	0g
Sodium	40mg	200mg

Nutrition information

The *per serve* column is handy for estimating how much you should eat.

One tablespoon of this dressing will add a large 11 grams of fat to your daily tally, so if you're on a low-fat diet (40–50 grams a day) a tablespoon of this dressing is one-fifth of your day's intake! You may want to use less or swap to a fat-free dressing. The good news is you only get two grams of saturated fat, the 'bad' fat for cholesterol and you'll get almost no protein, carbohydrate or fibre and a only small amount of salt (40 mg sodium).

The *Per 100ml* column helps you to compare products.

The figures in the *per 100ml* column are percentages. The 55 grams of fat listed means over half of this dressing is made fat of (55%), as you'd expect. Some dressings can be as high as 80 per cent fat, while fat-free dressing will have 0 per cent.

Why don't all food products have Nutrition Information Panels?
Some products are exempt from having to supply nutritional information. These include:
- Very small packages and foods like herbs, spices, salt, tea and coffee.
- Single ingredient foods, such as fresh fruit, vegetables, water and vinegar.
- Food sold at fundraising events.
- Food sold unpackaged (if a nutritional claim is not made).
- Food made and packaged at the point of sale (like sandwiches or fast food).

Step 4: Checking for allergens

Some ingredients, such as peanuts, seafood, fish, gluten, milk, soya beans and eggs can trigger allergic reactions and so are declared on the label. Even to the extent of informing the buyer that—while these ingredients are not part of the food in question—the food was manufactured in premises where these allergy triggering foods are processed.

Step 5: Do the claims stack up?

No added sugar
The product must not contain any added sugar, but may contain its own natural sugars (say from fruit or milk).

Reduced-fat salt
There should be at least a 25% reduction from the original product.

Low-fat
Must contain less than 3% fat for solid foods (1.5% for liquid foods).

fat-free
Must have less than 0.15% fat.

Nutrition claims that you need to check
Some manufacturers make claims to attract your attention, but beware! They can be misleading.

- The term 'light' (or 'lite') doesn't necessarily mean that the product is low in fat or kilojoules. Light could refer to a lighter texture, colour or taste of the product. For example: light olive oil.
- 'No cholesterol' or 'cholesterol free' on foods derived from plants, like margarine and oil, are meaningless because plant foods contain virtually no cholesterol anyway. Some, however, can be high in fat such as nuts and avocados.
- 93% fat-free means it still contains 7% fat but sounds 'low-fat'.
- 'Baked not fried' sounds healthier but could still have as much fat as fried items, so check the label *and* check to see how much of the fat is saturated!

What's the difference between a use-by-date and a best-before-date?
Foods with a shelf life of less than two years must carry a *best-before-date*. Foods that should not be consumed after a certain date for safety reasons must have a *use-by-date* and cannot be sold after that date. Generally use-by-dates are found on perishables such as meat, fish and dairy products.

Some foods carry the date they were manufactured or packed instead of a *use-by-date* so you can tell how fresh the food is. Breads and meats are often labelled with a *Baked on* or *Packed on* date.

For more nutrition information, visit Catherine Saxelby's website at: *www.foodwatch.com.au*

INDEX TO DELICIOUS LIVING